Combating Sleep Disorders

Combating Sleep Disorders

Kathy Sexton-Radek, PHD, CBSM
and Gina Graci, PHD, CBSM

Foreword by Phyllis C. Zee, MD, PHD

PRAEGER

Westport, Connecticut
London

Library of Congress Cataloging-in-Publication Data

Sexton-Radek, Kathy.
   Combating sleep disorders / Kathy Sexton-Radek and Gina Graci ;
foreword by Phyllis C. Zee.
        p. cm.
   Includes index.
   ISBN 978–0–275–98973–6 (alk. paper)
1. Sleep disorders—Popular works.   I. Graci, Gina.   II. Title.
   RC547.S47   2008
   616.8'498—dc22   2007048774

British Library Cataloguing in Publication Data is available.

Library of Congress Catalog Card Number: 2007048774
ISBN: 978–0–275–98973–6

First published in 2008

Praeger Publishers, 88 Post Road West, Westport, CT 06881
An imprint of Greenwood Publishing Group, Inc.
www.praeger.com

Printed in the United States of America

The paper used in this book complies with the
Permanent Paper Standard issued by the National
Information Standards Organization (Z39.48–1984).

10 9 8 7 6 5 4 3 2 1

I thank my patients for the privilege and trust they gave me as I set out to solve their sleep troubles. I wish to thank the Elmhurst College Library Staff, particularly Kathy Willis, Jennifer Paliatka, Donna Goodwyn, and Elaine Fetyko-Page for their resourceful assistance. Also, many thanks to Peggy Dumas for her word processing expertise. And, to my sons Brett, Neal, and Ted, my husband, Matt, and my mom, Helene, thank you for your support.
—*Kathy Sexton-Radek*

All my love and gratitude to my parents, Mary and Joseph, and my sister, Mary, for all their love, support, and encouragement.
—*Gina Graci*

Contents

Figures and Tables

FIGURES

TABLES

Foreword

Unfortunately, too many people accept sleeping poorly. Most do not know why they have sleep problems or how to solve them, and their struggles continue for far too long. This unique book by Doctors Kathy Sexton-Radek and Gina Graci will help explain and solve sleep problems in a straightforward, step-by-step, scientifically based approach. The field of sleep medicine is young, yet the practices of detecting and treating sleep disturbance have advanced at an accelerated rate. These authors are setting the pace by writing a book that is practical and much needed.

What makes this book so unique is that it serves two purposes: It is the first of its kind to act as an accompaniment for someone working with a sleep doctor, and it can help anyone wanting to know more about detecting sleep disturbance and ways to treat the disturbance. In a perfect world, every sleep doctor would like to be available for all the questions and answers that patients may have. This book provides the reader with answers, so if someone is working with a sleep doctor, he or she will have more insight prior to the first visit and during and throughout treatment, which can save both time and money.

Doctors Sexton-Radek and Graci first educate the reader about sleep, both from a scientific perspective and a layman's approach, and then ask the reader to become his own detective by looking at behaviors that may contribute to poor sleep and providing ways to change these behaviors so that sleep is no longer a struggle. What I find most impressive and unique is that these sleep specialists write about a model of change for promoting sleep change and maintenance of sleep over time. This model is a step-by-step account of what is needed at each stage to promote sleep change. The ultimate goal is to have a lasting effect on sleep—no more sleepless nights!

Together, Doctors Sexton-Radek and Graci have teamed up to create a novel, much-needed addition to the field of sleep medicine. *Combating Sleep Disorders* goes beyond self-help books; it specifically guides the reader in a logical, optimistic, step-by-step manner and provides resources for further work. Of particular importance are chapters 6 and 7, "Change Your Mind about Your Sleep" and "Alternative Treatments for Sleep." Here, the reader is furnished with all the how-tos to improve sleep and ways to change not just thoughts and behaviors but also lifestyle to promote better sleep.

The authors' credentials are ideal. Dr. Sexton-Radek has spent her career in researching and treating sleep disorders and has extensive written and published works. She is a licensed clinical psychologist and allied medical staff member at Suburban Pulmonary and Sleep Associates/Hinsdale Hospital. Dr. Graci is a well-known cancer and sleep disorder specialist and a certified behavioral sleep medicine specialist focusing on the evaluation and treatment of insomnia, specifically, problems with initiating and maintaining sleep.

If someone has encountered poor sleep, this book was written for that person. It is readable and focused and different from any sleep book ever written. The sleep disturbed have a choice to stop the sleepless nights.

                                                    Phyllis C. Zee, MD, PhD

Preface

This book is intended for readers experiencing poor sleep who are in treatment or plan to attend treatment from a sleep specialist. Sleep is often an overlooked necessity, and when we do not replenish our bodies with restful sleep, many physical and emotional complaints can result. Often, our own behaviors contribute to our sleep disturbance. We have become our own worst enemies, in terms of sleep functioning, because the bedroom often becomes a place of worrying, working, problem solving, watching television, reading, eating, and so forth, and it has lost its feeling of sanctuary and safe haven. These activities and behaviors can be incompatible with sleep and can delay sleep onset and help maintain wakefulness after waking from sleep.

With this change in behaviors, it is not surprising that the most common complaint of sleep disturbance is difficulty falling or staying asleep, generally referred to as insomnia. These sleep complaints result in people experiencing insufficient sleep and waking up feeling unrefreshed. *Combating Sleep Disorders* allows the reader to be guided in a stepwise manner, with each chapter furthering the reader's understanding of his own sleep and potential contributors to poor sleep.

This book also includes chapter highlights noted as *sleep notes* that may be useful tools in preparing the reader for meeting with a sleep specialist. These chapter deduction sections may also serve as helpful discussion points that the reader can choose to discuss during her sleep appointment. Additionally, this book also contains a standard sleep survey used by sleep professionals that the reader may want to consider if she feels her poor sleep may be attributable to other medical, psychological, environmental, or behavioral factors. Also, a list of resources is provided (i.e., general bibliography, Internet resources, and directories) to assist in helping the reader solve her sleep problems.

We hope this book serves to establish the belief and provide guidance in the concept that everyone can solve their sleep problems and restore natural sleep patterns.

Kathy Sexton-Radek, PhD, CBSM and
Gina Graci, PhD, CBSM

Section One
Understanding Sleep Medicine

CHAPTER 1

Signs of Poor Sleep

Sleep is defined as a series of complex, natural physiological rhythms. The National Sleep Foundation (NSF) estimates that we spend one-third of our lives sleeping.[1] We achieve the sleep that we do based on our need for sleep and the time of night when we get sleepy. Is sleep just determined by physiological events? No, behaviors also influence sleep patterns. Depending on what these behaviors are, they can actually interfere with or promote sleep.

We have allowed a flurry of responsibilities and obligations to impede upon our sleep time. From a physiological perspective, it does not take much to induce sleep, yet our sleep is being thwarted by our voluntary activities and behaviors (e.g., venti-size coffees that are consumed at varying times during the day and evening, Internet surfing, socializing); these behaviors accentuate the extended wakefulness.[2] Additionally, our student population tends to condense class schedules to accommodate full-time work schedules in conjunction with a busy social calendar. Teens and children have also extended the wake day to include homework, athletics, and Internet use. Taken together, record numbers of children, teens, young adults, adults, and the elderly are living each day in a sleep-deprived state. Why is sleep deprivation such a big concern? Results of a Gallup poll reported that 56 percent of the adult population reported daytime drowsiness as a problem. In that grouping, 31 percent stated that they had fallen asleep at the wheel at least once in their lifetime. Sleep deprivation is a very serious threat to safety and overall emotional and physical well-being. This accumulation of sleep loss does not dissipate; it does, however, reduce our capacity to function.[3,4]

To summarize, we should ask ourselves, "What are my chosen daily and evening activities or behaviors that shorten sleep, and what effects does shortened sleep have on my life?" The most likely outcome is excessive daytime sleepiness resulting in personality changes (e.g., irritability), memory and concentration difficulties, safety concerns (employment and automobile accidents), and an overall decrement in quality of life.

Unfortunately, we have become used to reducing our sleep time and/or experiencing fragmented sleep, which is not optimal. It is simply not healthy. The sleepiness felt day in and day out accumulates over time, resulting in poor functioning and reduced quality-of-life ratings. For example, a person is more likely to become irritable and moody when sleep deprived compared to someone who experiences restorative sleep on a daily basis.

After reading this far, the reader may ask, "What is my next step in solving my sleep problems?" This book will provide the how-tos to alter and improve daily and nighttime sleep patterns. The how-tos are easily explained and illustrated to assist in working independently or with a sleep specialist to guide the reader through a short-term course of behavior changes. The end result will be deeper sleep, more restful sleep, and more alertness and energy during the day.

Let us begin with ways of identifying and determining signs of poor sleep. First, rate (by taking a weekly average) how sleepy you feel during the week. A standard scale used in this area is called the Epworth Sleepiness Scale, which has been psychometrically tested and validated (figure 1.1).[5] Add up your ratings for each item, which will yield your total score. Your total score reflects a rating of sleepiness or intensity of sleepiness during waking hours. Scores can range from 0 to 21, with a score of 10 or higher denoting sleepiness of clinical significance.

Intuition may also serve in this type of assessment. Specifically, consider what time of day and what type of activities result in feeling sleepy. You may also include some other *context cues*. For example, when do you feel you need another cup of coffee, to get up to stretch your legs, the need to rub your eyes? Yes to all of these cues would result in a conclusion that you are perhaps sleepy. Feeling as if you are zoning out is a reminder of how lack of sleep impacts our lives.

Figure 1.1
Epworth Sleepiness Scale

Would you fall asleep in these situations? Use rating scale:

Never	Slight	Moderate	High
0-------------1-------------2-------------3			

1. Sitting and reading   ____

2. Watching TV   ____

3. Sitting, inactive in a public place   ____

4. As a passenger in a car riding for an hour without a break   ____

5. Lying down to rest in the afternoon when circumstances permit   ____

6. Sitting and talking with someone   ____

7. Sitting quietly after a lunch without alcohol   ____

8. In a car, while stopped for a few minutes in traffic   ____

In addition to sleepiness, the quality and quantity of sleep must also be addressed. Ratings of *poor, good,* or *excellent* or *light, fair,* or *deep* are some ways to describe how quality and quantity of sleep may be classified. If your sleep is disturbed, you are more likely to rate the quality of your sleep as poor, and if you are sleeping less than your ideal number of hours of sleep, you are most likely going to rate your quantity of sleep as poor. If you do not know the number of hours your body requires for restorative sleep, there is an easy way to figure it out. Think back to the last time you took a vacation. Ignore the first few nights of sleep (it is generally catch-up sleep), what was the length of your sleep? Generally, this question is a good heuristic to follow to determine your personal sleep need. In summary, if you experience less than good or fair sleep on a consistent basis, you most likely will experience excessive daytime sleepiness.

TOWARD AN UNDERSTANDING OF SLEEP

Approximately fifty-five years ago, sleep used to be thought of as a "dormant state of passive activity or no consequence."[2] This period of "no consequence" was hypothesized to serve as a much-needed downshifting in physiological activity from the day's events. We know much more today, however, especially with the burgeoning of sleep medicine, especially in regard to diagnosis, assessment, and treatment of sleep disorders. Sleep is considered now to be an active state of being; the mind is a 24-hour mind, and it does stop working, a surprising fact of which we often are not aware. We spend roughly one-third of our lives sleeping in this active state. Although the specific function of sleep still eludes researchers, many substantiated theories point to the necessity of good-quality sleep to our existence and overall well-being.

Different brain cell chemicals and neurotransmitters regulate our sleep-wake states by acting on a variety of cells in the brain.

Sleep-wake functioning is analogous to a light switch with on and off features. A type of switch setting systematically turns on sleep, including turning on different types of sleep (e.g., stages 1–4 and dream sleep), and systematically turns off each sleep stage correspondingly. This switch setting easily explains how our sleep progresses from light sleep to deep sleep and then transcends to dream, or REM, sleep. The neurochemical signaling begins when we fall asleep. An exact sleep chemical is still considered to be controversial, yet a number of studies suggest adenosine (a nucleoside) binds to cells and causes a cascade of events that promote drowsiness.[5] Adenosine levels in the blood increase during waking hours and have a cumulative effect throughout the day, causing drowsiness. During sleep, adenosine levels decline (unbind to cells), promoting wakefulness toward the end of the nocturnal period.[6] The cycle begins again once we are awake. It is not surprising that stimulants such as caffeine cause wakefulness because caffeine competes for the same receptors to which adenosine binds. If more receptors have caffeine bound to them, sleepiness is less likely to happen.

A REVIEW OF THE SLEEP STAGES

Sleep architecture refers to the various stages in the sleep-wake cycle, typically defined by a brainwave (EEG) recording. In healthy individuals without sleep problems, these stages occur in a regular pattern throughout a 24-hour period. Sleep is of two types, dream or rapid eye movement (REM) sleep that occurs every 1.5 hours throughout the sleep interval, or 18 percent to 25 percent of the sleep period.[7,8] REM periods vary from a number of minutes to an hour or more. REM sleep has a characteristic physiological pattern distinguished by the lateral saccadic (left to right) rhythm of the eyes, absence of muscle movement (atonia), and heightened cardiovascular arousal. Studies of the REM period by self-report have revealed the changing themes from everyday events to surreal wish fantasies toward the end of the sleep period.

In contrast, non-REM (NREM) sleep occupies a greater portion of the sleep period. NREM is further subdivided into stages 1, 2, 3, and 4, with corresponding physiological activity to each. Stage 1 is considered light sleep and is estimated to be approximately 5 percent of the sleep period. Stage 2 sleep is about 60 percent of the sleep interval and is considered formally to be sleep. Stages 3 and 4 sleep are often collapsed together and are classified as deep sleep, a physiological event characterized by slow brain wave patterns and increased immune system activity. Non-REM makes up approximately 10 percent to 15 percent of the sleep period.

A night of sleep is characterized as a predicted pattern beginning with the initiation of sleep onset (Stage 1) and progression to Stages 2, 3, and 4. Within 90 minutes after sleep onset, the first REM episode (generally four to five REM episodes per night) occurs. Following this sleep period, the cycle repeats itself, with at least four cycles of sleep per night. An excess or deficit in the amount of a type of sleep (e.g., no REM), a misordering of the timing of sleep (e.g., sleep begins with REM), or an intrusion into sleep represent conditions for further study to determine if a sleep disorder exists.

FUNCTION OF SLEEP

Sleep is needed for survival.[4] In animal studies, sleep-deprived rats subjected to extended periods of sleep loss developed disease and illness, with some resulting in death.[5] What does sleep loss do to our bodies? Our immune system becomes less efficient and productive with reduced sleep.[5,9] Our ability to fight off infection under increased stress levels can become compromised.

For instance, increased reports of cold- and flu-like symptoms are reported at college health clinics in response to surveys about high stress-response levels (commonly presented as sleep loss).[3] It is during deep (Stage 4) sleep when our immune system regenerates. Stage 4 sleep is also the time when growth hormone (the hormone responsible for growth and metabolism) is released, thus implicating the importance of a good night's sleep for children.

PROBLEM SLEEPINESS

The biological systems of our body follow a natural rhythm of activity and rest.[10] Many of these rhythms (cycles) are activated during the stages of sleep, usually deep sleep (Stages 3 and 4) or dream (REM) sleep. Overall, all cycles follow an approximate 24-hour schedule; hence the term *circadian* (i.e., "about a day") is used. When an individual's 24-hour schedule becomes skewed or altered due to work, travel, or personal habits, the timing of the sleep in terms of bedtime and wake time is offset. For instance, when traveling across time zones, we will experience a change in our sleep schedule.[11] This change may present as either a delay (sleep occurs at a later time) or advancement (sleep occurs at an earlier time) in our sleep time. Last, our natural drive for sleep is strongest during the day (A.M.) and nighttime (P.M.) between the hours of 1:00 and 4:00. This feeling of sleepiness that occurs during the hours between 1:00 P.M. and 4:00 P.M. is often misinterpreted as sleepiness resulting from having lunch.

Taken together, problem sleepiness occurs if we alter our schedule of activity and sleep at a time when the drive for sleepiness is the strongest. Treatment efforts address this change or desynchronization of our normal wake-sleep rhythms by scheduling naps, implementing light physical activity to the schedule and utilizing light therapy at varying times during the day to promote either sleepiness or wakefulness.

WHAT SLEEPINESS MEANS

We are generally aware of our level and ratings of sleepiness. We are all familiar with stories of businesspeople traveling and staying up late to prepare for a big presentation. Or there is the scenario of young adults and teens altering their sleep schedules with in-house socializing (e.g., instant messaging) by staying up into the late hours of the night. Additional examples include patients who are recovering from medical procedures who may easily awaken from experiencing pain or restlessly shifting positions while dipping in and out of sleep during the night. In each of these scenarios, poor sleep is experienced, and if these sleep patterns remain unabated, the individual is at risk for mood alterations and performance and health consequences.

A mounting sleep debt—regardless of the process that triggered it—has the same result: decreased performance efficiency, mood instability, and poor health and disease and disorder formation.[10] Our defensive response to the challenges we face with poor sleep is weakened and remains that way. Poor sleep, especially when continuously experienced, lowers the immune system response. Couple poor sleep with exposure to environmental toxins, disease and infection exposure, and/or mental or physical stress, and we may see how the immune system can significantly be lowered.

It could be argued that the most common signs of sleepiness are not just ignored; rather, we do not know how to detect these signs.[12] These signs are commonly reported as feeling the need to close the eyes, experiencing sensations of relaxed muscles, reduction in breathing (it starts to slow down), restless legs, and feeling chilled.[13] Ultimately, daytime sleepiness is the consequence of poor, short sleep.

To conclude, we ask you one question, "How sleepy are you?" To find the answer to this question, complete the Stanford Sleepiness Scale[14,15] (figure 1.2). If you are scheduled to see a sleep specialist, do not forget to bring these results with you to your visit.

Figure 1.2
Stanford Sleepiness Scale

Time	Naps (Length)	Sleepiness	Activity
6 a.m.			
7 a.m.			
8 a.m.			
9 a.m.			
10 a.m.			
11 a.m.			
12 p.m.			
1 p.m.			
2 p.m.			
3 p.m.			
4 p.m.			
5 p.m.			
6 p.m.			
7 p.m.			
8 p.m.			
9 p.m.			
10 p.m.			
11 p.m.			
12 a.m.			

Stanford Sleepiness Scale
Please mark the number that best describes your state of sleepiness once each hour.

1 – Feeling active and vital; alert, wide awake.
2 – Functioning at a high level, but not at peak; able to concentrate.
3 – Relaxed; awake; not at full alertness; responsive.
4 – A little foggy; not at peak; let down.
5 – Fogginess; beginning to lose interest in remaining awake; slowed down.
6 – Sleepiness; prefer to be lying down; fighting sleep; woozy.
7 – Almost in reverie; sleep onset soon; must struggle to remain awake.

Activity Level
First: List activity you are doing (i.e., sitting and thinking)
Second: Circle the number corresponding to the degree of physical energy involved next to the activity listed.

```
├──────┼──────┼──────┼──────┤
 1      2      3      4      5
None         Moderate     Excessive
      Little          Much
```

Sleep Notes

- We are chronically sleep deprived.
- Loss of sleep means loss of opportunity to other biological cycles and systems in our body, such as the immune system, to perform their biological role.
- Sleepiness is the brain's demand for sleep.
- How sleepy are you? Behavioral performance decrements have been found in sleep-deprived study participants.
- Bring completed Epworth and Stanford Sleepiness Scales to your appointment with your sleep specialist.

REFERENCES

1. National Sleep Foundation. (March, 2004). Sleep and America Poll. Washington, DC.
2. Sexton-Radek, K. (2004). *Sleep quality in young adults.* New York: Mellon Press.
3. Engle-Friedmen, M., Riela, S., Golan, R., Venteneac, A. M., Davis, C., Jefferson, A., et al. (2003). The effect of sleep loss on next day effect. *Journal of Sleep Research, 12,* 113–124.done
4. Coren, S. (1996). *Sleep thieves: An eye-opening exploration into the science and mysteries of sleep.* New York: Free Press.
5. Chokroverty, S. (1999). *Sleep disorders medicine: Basic science, technical considerations, and clinical aspects.* Boston: Butterworth Heinemann.
6. Johns, M. W. (1991). A new method of measuring daytime sleepiness: The Epworth Sleepiness Scale. *Sleep, 14,* 540.
7. Graci, G. M. (2005, September–October). Pathogenesis and management of cancer-related insomnia. *The Journal of Supportive Oncology, 3*(5), 349–359.
8. Graci, G., & Sexton-Radek, K. (2005). Treating sleep disorders using cognitive behavioral therapy and hypnosis. In R. A. Chapman (Ed.), *The clinical use of hypnosis in cognitive behavior therapy: A practitioner's casebook* (p. 348). New York: Springer.

9.   Horne, J. (1988). *Why we sleep.* Oxford: Oxford University Press.

10. Monk, T. H. (1991). *Sleep, sleepiness and performance.* Chichester, UK: Wiley.

11. Notti, L. (1990). *Losing sleep: How your sleeping habits affect your life.* New York: Morrow.

12. Heon-Jeong, L., Kim, L., & Suh, K. (2003). Cognitive deterioration and changes of P330 during total sleep deprivation. *Psychiatry and Clinical Neuroscience, 57,* 490–496.

13. Staupi, C. (1985). *Why we nap: Evolution, chronobiology and functions of polyphasic and ultrashort sleep.* Boston: Birkhauser.

14. Hoddes, E., Dement, W. C., & Zarcone, V. (1972). The development and use of the Stanford Sleepiness Scale (SSS). *Psychophysiology, 9,* 150.

15. Hoddes, E., Zarcone, V., Smythe, H., Phillips, R., & Dement, W. C. (1973). Quantification of sleepiness: A new approach. *Psychophysiology, 10,* 431.

CHAPTER 2

Sleep Loss Effects

Overstimulation in Americans from the activities we engage in instead of sleeping may be related to our poor sleep.[1] The popularity of activities that hinder sleep that we commonly engage in contribute to our sleep disturbances. Furthermore, a cover story of *New Scientist* (February 2006) discusses the increased percentage of the use of medicines to fall asleep as well as those that are used during the day to maintain wakefulness and alertness.[1] Research in this area is still under investigation, but there is an increased percentage of medication usage to extend wakefulness, induce sleep, lengthen the amount of deep sleep, increase alertness, and decrease the awareness of sleepiness.[1]

Knowing that more people are relying on medications for sleep and wakefulness, what is your sleep schedule and what are your sleep habits? Ask yourself the following questions:

- Under what conditions is it difficult to sleep?
- At what time during the night is it difficult to sleep?
- How many times during the night do you wake up?

- What wakes you up?
- How often do you have problems sleeping?

Also be aware of any sleepiness you feel in the daytime, your bedtime and wake time, and periods when you expect to be awake.[2] Note how any or all of these answers affect your ability to function and enjoy life. Here are some additional questions to help you understand how your sleep affects you:

- Having difficulty concentrating or making decisions?
- Experiencing drowsiness when you drive or are engaged in other activities?
- Feeling moody or irritable with others?

These questions are just examples used to illustrate the importance of sleep and how lack of sleep can affect our mental/cognitive abilities, personality, mood, and safety.

Now that we have explored the impact of sleep on our overall well-being, it is important to discuss how our body regulates sleep. Sleepiness is physiologically regulated by the following two primary processes:

1. The body's *circadian rhythm* causes an increase in sleepiness twice during a 24-hour period (in general, between midnight and 7:00 A.M. and in the midafternoon between 1:00 P.M. and 4:00 P.M.)
2. The *physiological need for sleep,* which is increased by sleep loss and sleep disruption.

The need for sleep and the circadian rhythm interact to determine the level of sleepiness and alertness.

The body needs these two processes to initiate sleep and to remain asleep. There are multiple factors, however, that can physically and psychologically prevent us from falling asleep.

Our muscles need to relax so that muscle tone in our head and neck and other regions of the body is at its most natural relaxed state, and our breathing patterns change (become slower) during different stages of wakefulness and sleep. Physiologically, we also need to have comfortable temperature and noise levels as well as being free from thirst, hunger, pain, or physical discomfort. In summary, if environmental and physiological conditions are not conducive to sleep, in terms of temperature, heart rate, noise, light, and physical comfort, then sleep is less likely to happen.

Additionally, psychological reasons are the most common explanations for experiencing difficulty falling asleep and the ability to maintain sleep. There are different primary regions in the brain that control sleep stages and the maintenance of sleep. One of the regions is the frontal lobe, where thinking, problem solving, analyzing, and worrying occur. Other regions of the brain, including the back of the brain (specifically the brain stem), are responsible for activating and terminating sleep stages. In summary, engaging in mentally stimulating activities (frontal lobe) and trying to elicit sleep (brain stem) are simply incompatible. It is impossible to think, solve problems, analyze, and/or worry while falling asleep or during sleep; these are mentally stimulating activities. You can give yourself permission to turn off your brain at night, but just for the night, because you will be able to return your attention to these activities during the next day. It is recommended that you make notes, create a list, or compose reminder messages of things pending or things of importance to you at least two hours before bedtime. These reminder or problem lists will assist you in clearing your mind and help you achieve falling asleep and staying in a deep sleep.

The prevalence rates for sleep disturbance are high because sleep is very sensitive to stress and emotional upset. Major life events and minor life events that accumulate negatively impact our sleep. We spend increased amounts of time problem solving, analyzing, and worrying, and these behaviors often intrude on our nighttime sleep. We spend time in bed engaging in these behaviors, which are mentally stimulating behaviors and fragment or disrupt our sleep. In addition to psychosocial stressors, lifestyle factors also play a role. For instance, changes in lifestyle factors such as transitioning from being employed full-time to becoming a part-time worker or a student transitioning to full-time employment requiring early-morning schedule changes can affect our sleep. Furthermore, we have to consider the full-time worker who works daily from 9:00 to 5:00 and retires and has to adjust her schedule to new and differing activities (such as playing golf once a week or fixing things around the house). This transition in lifestyle or daily activities can be stressful because it can be unfamiliar. Sleep disturbance may occur when schedules change, especially in the case of individuals retiring, because these individuals often do not have activities to occupy their day and instead may fill their day with resting or taking naps, and these behaviors affect nighttime sleep.

One of the most basic sensations of sleep loss is a profound sense of sleepiness. We know that sleep is necessary for our bodily systems to work efficiently. Too little sleep makes us feel cloudy, inattentive, uninterested, and irritable, and we may experience difficulty with concentration.[2] It also leads to impaired memory and physical performance.

You do not have to experience complete sleep deprivation to feel the significant effects of sleep loss on psychological and physical well-being. Partial sleep loss may take the effect of occasionally losing a good night's sleep. Having frequent awakenings during the night may also result in experiencing the effects of partial sleep loss that detrimentally affects our quality of life.

If we abbreviate our nighttime sleep, resulting in insufficient sleep, we experience partial sleep loss with the consequence of prolonging a chronic state of sleep loss. This chronic state of sleep loss can have serious penalties on cognitive[2,3] and physical functioning. In addition to the quality of life decrements, there are also a number public health and safety accidents that occur due to loss of alertness and sustained attention. Sustained attention is absolutely necessary when operating heavy industrial machinery or participating in complicated procedures involving dangerous machinery, such as construction machine operation. All are quite dangerous for the partially sleep-deprived individual because it places that person and others at risk.

Self-report measures completed in a census fashion demonstrate that a larger percentage of individuals with compromised sleep also report health problems.[4,5,6] A greater percentage of these individuals are involved in accidents at work or also report experiencing employment difficulties. Although there is no clear cause and effect, we know that these individuals report a greater incidence of sleep problems compared to a control group.

WHEN SLEEPINESS BECOMES A PROBLEM: A SYMPTOM OF DISORDER

Insomnia, the most common sleep disorder, has significant negative consequences on quality of life. [7,8,9] These consequences are primarily due to the effects of total or partial sleep loss on our overall well-being. It is also hypothesized that insomnia might actually be due to another type of sleep disorder.[10,11] For instance, undiagnosed obstructive sleep apnea patients often report experiencing significant sleep loss and may report difficulty falling asleep after an awakening. Scientists and sleep specialists in this area diagnose sleep disorders using a consensus of more than eighty conditions, and in many of those, insomnia might be a symptom rather than the actual sleep difficulty.

INSOMNIA

Insomnia is a complex, multifaceted complaint that may involve difficulties falling asleep, staying asleep, early-morning awakenings (with an inability to return to sleep), and/or a complaint of non-refreshing sleep that produces significant impairment.[12,13,14,15] The most prominent feature of insomnia remains the complaint of poor sleep, either of inadequate duration or quality, which impacts quality of life, mood, energy, and daytime functioning.[16,17] An insomnia complaint almost always involves some type of increased arousal state.

The two most common types of insomnia disorders (not including insomnia associated with a medical disorder) are *adjustment* and *psychophysiological* sleep disorders.[13] Adjustment sleep disorder is a condition in which an individual has experienced a significant life stressor (such as death of a loved one or being diagnosed with a life-threatening illness) that interferes with sleep. This type of sleep disturbance is more commonly associated with a transient sleep disturbance and generally abates within one month.[13] When this type of transient insomnia does not attenuate over time, however, it can progress to chronic insomnia, often accompanied by depression. In comparison, psychophysiological insomnia is a sleep disorder that results from the presence of heightened arousal in which *somatized* tension and learned sleep-preventing associations (e.g., nervousness, anxiety, ruminative thoughts) interfere with nocturnal sleep.[12]

People's faulty beliefs and attitudes about sleep and sleep disturbance are significant factors in continuing sleep problems.[13] Many people believe that eight hours of continuous sleep each night is necessary to maintain daily functioning; however, there is wide variability in nightly sleep patterns. Further, there appears to be no evidence that occasional loss of sleep has any lasting effect. Nevertheless, sleep disturbance often elicits anxiety about continued sleep disturbance, leaving patients lying in bed worrying about whether they will get to sleep or get enough sleep in the coming night. This kind of worry and anxiety further contributes to maintaining that disturbance. Of course, the continuing use of maladaptive sleep behaviors, including an excessive amount of time in bed, napping, and an irregular sleep-wake cycle, will both maintain and possibly worsen sleep disturbances.[13]

OBSTRUCTIVE SLEEP APNEA

The most common reason that people are referred to a sleep clinic outside of insomnia is for obstructive sleep apnea. Sleep apnea is a sleep-related breathing disorder and is a very treatable sleep disorder. Patients with sleep apnea may complain about having difficulty maintaining sleep, experiencing daytime sleepiness, and having ruminative thoughts centering on lack of sleep.[8] This complaint could easily lead to a diagnosis and treatment for insomnia. Insomnia treatment most likely will fail, however, because the patient's reported difficulty with maintaining sleep is associated with physiological factors responsible for the disordered breathing that occurs while sleeping.

With sleep apnea, the individual stops breathing during sleep because the pharyngeal airway (area at the back of the throat) has narrowed and collapsed (due to excess tissue in the back of the throat, anatomical abnormalities, etc.), obstructing the airway (the hallmark feature of obstructive sleep apnea), and the body awakens (an evolutionary adaptive response to protect the body) in order to restore breathing. When air is blocked from moving down the throat during the night, the body immediately transitions to a state of light sleep, which will awaken the body. The body awakens from receiving signals from the brain to "pull air through the nose and release it through the mouth."[1]

Snoring is generally a cardinal symptom of obstructive sleep apnea and is caused by excess tissue in the back of the throat that prematurely flaps as air is released through the mouth and vibrates. Snoring can also occur if this excess tissue is blocking the opening of the throat, and it is common to either hear a snort or gasp for air.

Individuals with sleep apnea seem to have characteristic features of snoring. The most prominent is the volume level that is often disruptive to bed partners. Arousal may or may not be associated with snoring or with sleep apnea events. The propensity to develop sleep apnea increases as people mature (e.g., gain weight) and in postmenopausal women when they lose estrogen, which served as a protective factor against sleep apnea. Postmenopausal women tend to gain weight, and this weight gain is a contributing factor for sleep-related breathing events. As individuals gain weight, there is an increase in adipose (fat) tissue, especially around the abdomen and in the throat areas, increasing the incidence of apnea or snoring events. Additionally, most individuals usually seek treatment for sleep disturbance when they are in adulthood; however, children can also be diagnosed with sleep apnea. It is less common than in adults and is treated differently. In adults, treatment for obstructive sleep apnea generally includes changes in lifestyle, weight reduction, cessation of smoking, and reduction of excessive alcohol use.

How is sleep apnea diagnosed? Obstructive sleep apnea can only be diagnosed using a polysomnogram (i.e., an overnight sleep study). A polysomnogram evaluates all aspects of sleep (e.g., brain waves, heart rhythms, lung functioning, blood oxygen levels, etc.) to determine if a person is experiencing the appropriate amounts and staging of sleep and to ensure that there is no medical reason (e.g., cardiac problems) interfering with sleep. If there are disturbances in sleep, the polysomnogram helps determine what the contributing factors to this disturbed sleep are.

If an individual meets the criteria for a diagnosis of obstructive sleep apnea, the gold standard is continuous positive airway pressure (CPAP). A CPAP mask is placed over the mouth and nose, which gently pushes humidified, warm air to the back of the throat at such a level that it stimulates the tissue to contract, keeping the opening clear and available for air exchange. Many sleep professionals equate CPAP treatment to a so-called pneumatic splint because it keeps the airway from collapsing during the sleep. CPAP uses room air rather than oxygen to stimulate and maintain the opening of the airway. Nasal dryness can occur (among a low percentage of users) and is generally treated by adding a humidification feature to the CPAP machine. If an individual complains that the CPAP pressure is troublesome, adding a ramping feature to the CPAP unit generally solves this complaint. Ramping features on CPAP machines control CPAP administration by beginning with very low pressures and slowly increasing the CPAP pressure until the appropriate pressure is attained. Generally, an individual will fall asleep before her targeted CPAP pressure is reached.

Since its development in the 1980s, the CPAP machine is one of the more widely distributed methods of treating moderate to severe sleep apnea.[1] Other medical approaches include surgical procedures to reduce or eliminate the excess pharyngeal tissue that is causing the obstructive apnea events or dental retainer devices that are custom made to move the lower jaw forward, allowing more space at the back of the throat to keep the airway open during sleep. Retainer devices are only worn at night and do not permanently move the jaw forward.

SLEEP DISTURBANCE IN TEENS AND ADULTS

Children and teens sleep differently than adults. As children mature into their teens and young adulthood, the long sleep periods are no longer observed, for the sleep period shortens to approximately the time of adult sleep (i.e., about seven hours). Young adults and teens are susceptible to sleep disorders. The most common are narcolepsy (disorder of excessive daytime sleepiness, sleep attacks, and muscle tone weakness), delayed sleep onset (inability to fall asleep before 1:00 A.M. to 2:00 A.M. and attributable to biological irregularities), and insomnia. Lifestyle factors are severely altered with these conditions, with below average satisfaction in one or more life areas.[18] Narcolepsy is treated with behavioral therapy of naps and medication.

Delayed sleep phase disorder, a category of circadian sleep disorders in which the timing of sleep is excessively delayed, is common in adolescents and young adults. This delay results from biological factors and not voluntary behaviors. The mechanisms responsible for sleep onset/initiation (e.g., hormones and neuro-chemicals) become faulty, resulting in the disruption of the timing of sleep (i.e., bedtimes become delayed—move forward in time—usually after the midnight hour). Sleep is delayed on a consistent basis. As a result of this delayed sleep initiation, individuals are compelled to sleep much later in the morning in order to acquire some sleep.[4] Consequently, the next night's sleep is again delayed because the individual is not tired at her regular bedtime, and this cycle keeps repeating itself.

When we have consistently set bedtime and wake-time sched-ules, our brains adapt to these sleep-wake cycles.[1,4] It is easy to understand how our behaviors impact our sleep and how these be-haviors can influence insufficient sleep, cause disturbed sleep, and change our sleep-wake schedules. For instance, the use of bright light (natural or with special lamps) is the number one regulator of sleep. Bright light stimulates a part of the brain (i.e., optic chias-matic nucleus, the sleep center of the brain) that regulates sleep.[1,2] Sleep-related hormones such as melatonin are released from the sleep center to assist in initiating and maintaining sleep.

Delayed sleep disorders must be differentiated from sleep pat-terns that mimic delayed sleep disorders that result from voluntary behaviors. When young adults experience irregularities in their sleep patterns that are due to voluntary behaviors, a diagnosis of delayed sleep disorder is not appropriate.[4] Sometimes, the onset of sleep is delayed by personal choice in order to conduct activities like American Online Instant Messenger (AIM), online chatting, playing video games, viewing DVDs, and general social activities. For instance, instead of sleeping, students try to balance their academic studies and/or employment with social activities. On average, both young adults and older adults try to accomplish just too much in a 24-hour period; the end result is delaying sleep, leading to insufficient sleep. If done on a regular basis, the brain adapts to this delayed or adjusted bedtime (most likely moving the bedtime forward two to four hours) as its regular bedtime, even though an individual's sleep need remains unaltered. For instance, if an individual requires eight hours of sleep to optimally function but reduces sleep time to six-and-a-half hours on a daily basis, the individual is consistently in a *sleep need* state due to insufficient sleep. The individual most likely will experience difficulty in trying to accomplish work or difficulty functioning in the early-morning, later-morning, or afternoon hours because of this voluntary delay in sleep onset. Young adults find it increasingly difficult to arise for a first-period class, to waken for work, to feel alert and ready for the day at the early-morning hour when they are in this pattern.

SLEEPINESS: HEALTH, PERFORMANCE, AND SAFETY FACTS

Sleepiness secondary to sleep deprivation can worsen medical diseases such as diabetes and epilepsy.[3,6] Mental health conditions, such as depression and anxiety, typically involve sleep disturbance (either sleeping too much [hypersomnia] or sleeping too little [insomnia]) as part of the symptom profile. Furthermore, in sleep restriction studies of undergraduates, mood, tension, and energy levels were found to be more affected with extreme sleep restriction schedules as compared to ad hoc schedules.[4] The self-reported changes in mood were reversed once participants returned to their regular sleep schedules. Additionally, behavioral studies of sleep (reducing or depriving dream [REM] sleep and measuring the impact on daytime behaviors) demonstrated a reduced ability to carry out math problems and an increase in short-term memory difficulties, along with attention and concentration impairments.[4]

Sleep deprivation, regardless of the causal factors (e.g., staying up late voluntarily or having sleep apnea), decreases levels of alertness and affects many areas of safety, especially driving. A massive health campaign to prevent driving accidents secondary to sleepiness (the highest rates are among teen drivers) is imperative. The National Sleep Foundation has begun this campaign to prevent dangerous situations for sleepy adults and teens (figure 2.1).

Figure 2.1
National Sleep Foundation driving while drowsy precautions

Driving while drowsy puts all of us at risk.

Are You at Risk?
Before you drive, check to see if you are:
- Sleep deprived or suffering from poor-quality sleep; six hours of sleep or less triples your risk.
- Driving long distances without proper rest breaks.
- Driving at night between midnight and 6:00 a.m. when you are normally asleep and during the midafternoon when there is a natural tendency to sleep.
- Driving alone or on a long, rural, dark or boring road.
- Taking medication that may cause sleepiness, such as cold tablets, antihistamines or antidepressants.
- Drinking even small amounts of alcohol.

DO
- Stop driving.
- Find a safe place to stop for a break or for the night.
- Pull off into a safe, well-lighted area away from traffic and take a brief nap; a minimum of 15 to 20 minutes is best.
- Drink coffee or another type of caffeine drink to promote short-term alertness if needed. (It takes about 30 minutes for caffeine to enter the bloodstream.) Caffeine is also available in soft drinks, chewing gum and tablets. Caffeine and a nap together offer short-term benefits.
- Get off the road if you hit shoulder rumble strips. These are deep grooves that are placed on high-speed roads to alert you when you are leaving the road.

Sleep Notes

- Loss of sleep means loss of opportunity for bodily biological cycles and systems, such as the immune system, to perform their roles.
- Sleepiness is the brain's demand for sleep.
- How sleepy are you? Behavioral, physical, and psychological functioning declines with sleep deprivation.

Chapter Exercises

1. Keep track of your sleep for two weeks. Note bedtime, wake-up time, number of awakenings, how long it took to fall asleep, how long you were awake during an awakening, and when you got out of bed in the morning.
2. Keep track (in your journal/daytime planner/personal digital assistant (PDA)) of the number of changes in your schedule that you made to accommodate your feelings of sleepiness. When and how often did you modify your schedule/lifestyle because of poor sleep?

REFERENCES

1. Nelson, G. (2006, February). Conquering sleep: Move over nature, we're taking control. *The New Scientist, Issue 2539,* 43–49.
2. Sexton-Radek, K. (1998). Pre-sleep autonomic arousal as a distinguishing factor of sleep pattern type. *Perceptual and Motor Skills, 87,* 261–262.
3. Dement, W. C., & Vaughn, C. (1999). *The promise of sleep.* New York: Random House.
4. Sexton-Radek, K. (2003). *Sleep quality in young adults.* New York: Mellon Press.
5. Coren, S. (1996). *Sleep thieves.* New York: Free Press Paperbacks/Simon and Schuster.

6. Johnson, M. P., Duffy, J. F., Dijk, D. J., Ronda, J. M., Dyal, C. M., & Czeisler, C. A. (1992). Short-term memory, alertness and performance: A reappraisal of their relationship to body temperature. *Journal of Sleep Research, 1,* 642–656.

7. Vgontza, A. (2006). Researchers gaining more understanding of sleep, sleep loss, daytime sleepiness and fatigue in healthy adults. *Science Daily.* Retrieved June 6, 2006, http://www.sciencedaily.com/releases/1999/08/998023071731.htm

8. Lee, H., Kim, L., & Suh, K. (2003). Cognitive deterioration and changes in P300 during total sleep deprivation. *Psychiatry and Clinical Neurosciences, 57,* 490–496.

9. Graci, G. M. (2005, September–October.). Pathogenesis and management of cancer-related insomnia. *The Journal of Supportive Oncology, 3*(5), 349–359.

10. Graci, G. M., & Hardie, J. C. (2006). Evidenced based hypnotherapy for the management of sleep disorders. *Journal of Clinical and Experimental Hypnosis* (manuscript accepted for publication).

11. Graci, G., & Sexton-Radek, K. (2005). Treating sleep disorders using cognitive behavioral therapy and hypnosis. In R. A. Chapman (Ed.), *The clinical use of hypnosis in cognitive behavior therapy: A practitioner's casebook* (p. 348). New York: Springer.

12. American Sleep Disorders Association Diagnostic Classification Steering Committee. (1997). *The international classification of sleep disorders: Diagnostic and coding manual.* Rochester, NY: American Academy of Sleep Medicine.

13. American Psychiatric Association. (1994). *Diagnostic and statistical manual of mental disorders* (4th ed.). Washington, DC: Author.

14. Savard, J., & Morin, C. M. (2001). Insomnia in the context of cancer: A review of a neglected problem. *Journal of Clinical Oncology, 19,* 895–908.

15. Edinger, J. D., Bonnet, M. H., Bootzin, R. R., Doghramji, K., Dorsey, C. M., Espie, C. A. et al. (2004). Derivation of research diagnostic criteria for insomnia: Report of an American Academy of Sleep Medicine work group. *Sleep, 27,* 1567–1596.

16. Morin, C. (1993). *Insomnia: Psychological assessment and management.* New York: Guilford Press.

17. Morin, C. M. (2000). The nature of insomnia and the need to refine our diagnostic criteria. *Psychosomatic Medicine, 62,* 483–485.

18. Sexton-Radek, K. (1982). Need satisfaction in narcolepsy. *Rehabilitation Literature, 43*(3–4), 82–85.

CHAPTER 3

Sleep Medicine Facts

This chapter describes what happens to our brains when sleep occurs. When we fall asleep, our brains allow us to experience an altered state of consciousness—if it is not tampered with—and we sleep. Sleep researchers have utilized brain measurement and body measurement techniques to establish parameters of sleep. From these measurements, we have a greater understanding of the appropriate timing, quantity, and quality of sleep. Your understanding of the basic science of sleep will assist you in making the necessary changes to improve your behaviors that impact your sleep. This basic understanding will also allow you to work more effectively with your sleep specialist.

Sleep researchers, utilizing brain wave (electroencephalogram, or EEG) patterns have been able to categorize different types of sleep patterns that reflect two basic types of sleep[1] (see chapter 1). The first one is called non-rapid eye movement (NREM) sleep. NREM sleep is characterized by varying levels of physiological activity that correspond to physiological (i.e., respiratory, cardiovascular) events.[1,2] The other type of sleep is called rapid eye movement (REM) sleep that is characterized by highly variable changes in physiological activity cycling between significant physiological activity (i.e., phasic) and no activity (tonic) periods.

Sleep architecture refers to the different sleep patterns (i.e., percentage of time spent in different sleep stages, the timing of sleep, and the pattern of our sleep stages) that characterize our sleep. For instance, it seems that when you fall asleep at night your body steps through an architecture of light sleep to increasingly deeper sleep only to wake up momentarily, after about an hour and a half, for another type of sleep, that is rapid eye movement sleep.[1] It is a specific and gradual stair-stepping pattern from light sleep to deep sleep that happens four times (or four cycles throughout the night). The majority of our NREM sleep occurs in Stage 2, totaling approximately 60 percent of our night. Stages 3 and 4 are sometimes called deep sleep. In Stage 1 sleep (light sleep), we are easily aroused, but this arousal state varies as we transition from Stage 1 to Stages 2, 3, and 4. These numbered stages correspond to deeper levels of sleep and difficulty of arousal. It is more difficult to awaken someone from Stage 4 sleep than it is from Stages 3, 2, or 1.[1,2]

As the brain transitions from Stage 1 to Stage 4 sleep, the body prepares itself for the next sleep stage, rapid eye movement (REM) sleep. It is called rapid eye movement sleep because there are specific periods during this sleep stage in which the eyes move from left to right.[3] It is also hypothesized that dreaming occurs during REM sleep. Time spent in REM sleep increases throughout the sleep period, with our greatest periods of REM sleep occurring in the early-morning hours. On average, we have four to five REM (dream) periods that last from a few moments to several minutes.

Dream content is characteristic of the time of night when the dream episode occurs. For instance, during the beginning of the sleep period (when NREM predominates), dreams typically involve recalling the day's events, things that are of importance, things accomplished, and things to accomplish for the next day.

In comparison, dreams change toward the end of the night (i.e., generally near awakening), when dreams are typically more florid and perceptual.

In summary, sleep generally consists of approximately four repetitions of sleep cycling from Stage 1 to Stages 3 and 4, with REM sleep occurring between these repetitions. Sleep onset generally begins at a regular time each night, and this predicted pattern of sleepiness is how we schedule our bedtimes. Similarly, our bodies have set waking times that will normally occur if there are no intrusions or alterations to these patterns of sleep.

It is common to need an alarm clock to awaken from sleep. This is in part due to our bodies' own demands for sleep but also reflecting our voluntary behaviors that interfere with sleep. Bedtimes and wake-up times in today's culture are more reflective of the importance we place on social demands and obligations than on providing our bodies with natural sleep needs.

SLEEP CHANGES ACROSS THE LIFE SPAN

Sleep constantly changes with aging. As we age, our sleep architecture changes in regard to the proportion and percentage of sleep obtained. For instance, as we advance in age, the amount of sleep that is needed is reduced by approximately 10 percent of what was needed during young adulthood.[4] The distribution of the amount and timing of sleep, as well as time spent in different sleep stages, changes throughout our life span.

NEWBORN SLEEP

Newborns have wonderful sleep that is initiated with REM sleep (unlike children and adults who begin sleep with NREM sleep), and they spend 50 percent of their sleep dreaming. As newborns mature, their sleep becomes more similar to adult sleep; that is, they initiate sleep with NREM. Additionally, deep sleep occurs at a greater extent with newborns and children. The release of growth hormone occurs at an accelerated rate during (and only during) deep sleep. Children correspondingly spend more time in deep sleep than adults. The essential feature is necessary for fundamental needs, such as healing, to larger-scale, longer-term needs, such as growth within the body or making ready for growth of bones within the body.

CHILDREN'S AND ADOLESCENTS' SLEEP

Children's and adolescents' sleep requires a separate discussion. When a child or adolescent is tired or sleepy because of a poor night's sleep, his or her behavior is likely to be expressed much differently than an adult who is sleepy.[5] Children and adolescents experience excessive activity rather than the symptoms of fatigue and withdrawal, which are commonly seen in adults.[3] The National Sleep Foundation provides information on the appropriate amounts of sleep based on a child's age as well as the appropriate bedtimes for children based on age (table 3.1).

Table 3.1
Children and Sleep: Helping Your Child
Develop Healthy Sleep Habits

How much sleep should my child get?	
Age	**Hours of Sleep**
0–2 months	16–18
2–12 months	14–15
1 year–3 years	12–14
3–5 years	11–13
5–12 years	10–11
Adolescence	9–10

Sleep is a vital need, essential to a child's health and growth. Sleep promotes alertness, memory, and performance. Children who get enough sleep are more likely to function better and are less prone to behavioral problems and moodiness. That is why it is important for parents to start early and help their children develop good sleep habits.

Each child is different and has different sleep needs. Table 3.1 presents *recommended* hours of sleep for children and adolescents. [5]

Helpful Tips

- Maintain a regular, consistent set bedtime.
- Create a presleep bedtime routine that is a positive and relaxing experience without interference from TV or videos. Save your child's favorite relaxing, nonstimulating activity or activities for right before bedtime; these activities should occur in the child's bedroom.
- Keep the bedtime environment (e.g., light, temperature) the same all night long.

Children explore their environment due to willingness or motivation to develop an understanding of this environment.[3] This motivation to learn may also promote resistance to bedtime behaviors because the child or adolescent may not always be able to discharge the activity or energy that accumulated during the day. On rare occasions, when this activity or energy cannot be discharged, behavioral and/or psychological problems may occur. Research findings have identified a high association between sleep disorders and psychiatric disorders in children and adolescents.[3] Neurobehavioral factors have been implicated in children with psychiatric disorders who are experiencing sleep disturbance.[1,3,5] These neurobehavioral factors include difficulty with attention, concentration, impulsivity, thinking, and memory.

Other causes of disrupted sleep in children or adolescents may be attributable to excessive limb movements or sleep-related breathing events; however, the most common disruption in child or adolescent sleep is a clinical diagnosis of obstructive sleep apnea. It is important to reiterate that children and adolescents do not express fragmented sleep due to sleep-disordered breathing events (apnea events) as adults do, thus it is not easily detected.[6]

It may be beneficial to have your child's tonsils or adenoids examined if he or she reports poor sleep or exhibits hyperactivity. A thorough ear, nose, and throat exam may reveal oversize tonsils or adenoids.[1,5] These oversize structures may obstruct breathing during sleep. The general treatment for sleep apnea caused by enlarged tonsils and/or adenoids is to have a tonsillectomy with or without adenoid removal. This procedure usually resolves the problem.

BEHAVIORAL INFLUENCES

Second to these health and medically related issues to poor sleep in children and adolescents are the behavioral influences.[4,6] For the stressed or anxious child or adolescent, bedtime can be threatening because it represents an unwanted time of separation from the parent(s) and from safe, familiar activities. Other behavioral factors resulting in disturbed sleep of children and adolescents are not engaging in enough physical activity or exercise, ear infection, atopic dermatitis, allergy medicine administered too close to bedtime, food allergies, irregular and/or extended napping, or hunger.[6,7,8] Once these behavioral factors are regulated, sleep is restored.

LIMIT SETTING DISORDERS

Children and adolescents commonly experience resistance to bedtime. This resistance can take on a variety of forms. Approximately 30 percent of parental requests to primary care providers are to treat bedtime behavioral problems.[4] It is not uncommon for children or adolescents to refuse to cooperate with presleep bedtime behaviors (e.g., bathing, engaging in calming activities) or when it is time to go to bed. Parents often engage in demanding and excessive rituals that include, but are not limited to, lying in bed with the child until he falls asleep or complying with children's requests for something to eat or drink. Behavioral problems are also likely to occur when parents or caregivers do not enforce a regular bedtime.

EVALUATION AND TREATMENT OF CHILDHOOD AND ADOLESCENT SLEEP DISTURBANCE

Sleep specialists will conduct specialized interviews, sometimes accompanied by psychological testing of children and adolescents with extreme sleep disturbance. It is not uncommon for an overnight sleep study (polysomnogram) to be conducted, followed by a daylong nap study.[1,5] These nighttime and daytime sleep studies are often ordered to rule out medical factors that may be influencing the disturbed sleep. Additionally, sleep specialists may also evaluate and treat a variety of childhood sleep disorders that may or may not present with behavioral factors. These sleep disorders include, but are not limited to, sleep apnea, sleep onset association disorder, limit setting sleep disorder, childhood insomnia, breathing-related problems, restless legs syndrome/periodic limb movement disorder, and circadian rhythm sleep disorder.[1,5,7]

Sleep Notes

- Sleep follows a natural pattern.
- The two types of sleep, non-rapid eye movement and rapid eye movement sleep, are distinct physical events that are measured by brain wave patterns.

Exercises

1. Study your sleep log and discuss your sleep functioning with your sleep specialist to determine what your sleep pattern is like; rate your sleep quality, how many hours are you sleeping on average per night, and what is your required number of hours of sleep to feel rested.

2. Can you identify some factors in your life and/or internal factors (biological or psychological) that may account for your poor sleep?

REFERENCES

1. Kryger, M. H., Roth, T., & Dement, W. C. (2006). *Principles and practices of sleep medicine* (4th ed.). New York: Elsevier.
2. Coren, S. (1996). *Sleep thieves.* New York: Free Press.
3. Dahl, R. (1996). The regulation of sleep and arousal: Development and psychopathology. *Development and Psychopathology, 8,* 3–27.
4. Sexton-Radek, K. (2003). *Sleep quality in young adults.* New York: Mellon Press.
5. Mindell, J. A. (2005). *Sleeping through the night: How infants, toddlers and their parents can get a good night's sleep.* New York: Harper Collins.
6. Chervin, R. D., & Archblood, K. H. (2001). Hyperactivity and polysomnographic findings in children evaluated for sleep-disturbed breathing. *Sleep, 24*(3), 313–320.
7. Owens, J. A., Spirito, A., & Marcotte, A. 2000). Neuropsychological and behavioral correlates of obstructive sleep apnea syndrome in children: A preliminary study. *Sleep and Breathing, 4*(2), 67–76.
8. Walters, A. S., Mandelbaum, D. E., Lewin, D. S,. Kugler, S., England S. J., & Miller, M. (2000). Dopaminergic therapy in children with restless legs/periodic limb movements in sleep and ADHD. *Pediatric Neurology, 22*(3), 182–186.

CHAPTER 4

How Sleep Is Measured

WHAT TO EXPECT FROM YOUR FIRST VISIT WITH A SLEEP SPECIALIST

In reading this book, you may be searching for an explanation of the process that has occurred for you already. That is to say, you may have already gone to see a sleep specialist about your sleep difficulties and are now trying to process what went on or what is going to happen. The treatment interventions for improving sleep (with the guidance of a sleep specialist) are effective. These interventions require commitment and involvement.

The purpose of the initial visit is to gather preliminary information. It is commonplace to be asked a standard set of questions. In fact, you may be asked about components of your sleep that you had already explained to your primary care provider or provided to your sleep specialist when you called to schedule an appointment. It is likely that you were asked about your sleep condition/functioning, and then you may have been e-mailed, faxed, or mailed some paper-and-pencil measures to complete and bring with you during your visit. The importance of gathering preliminary information prior to your office visit is essential for the establishment of an accurate diagnosis and administration of the appropriate treatment as well as the establishment of some baseline information that is used in evaluating the effectiveness of treatment.

OBJECTIVE MEASURES USED FOR OBTAINING DIAGNOSTIC INFORMATION

It is less common for an all-night sleep study, called a polysomnogram, to be requested by the physician. The objective measures commonly used for measuring nocturnal sleep are polysomnography recordings and actigraphy. PSG is not indicated for evaluation of transient insomnia, chronic insomnia, or insomnia associated with psychiatric disorders.[1] When a patient reports continued sleep disturbance (especially if the patient is elderly or lives alone) in the absence of contributing behavioral factors, however, a PSG is useful to determine the causal factors responsible for the sleep disturbance (e.g., obstructive sleep apnea, periodic leg movements, etc.).[2] A PSG recording monitors several variables, including brain wave activity, respiratory and cardiac functions, as well as blood-oxygen levels. PSG recordings allow for an in-depth look at all avenues of sleep and are the appropriate tool for diagnosing long-term sleep disorders. They also provide information about the ordering of stages of sleep and the general amount of time spent in each sleep stage, which is very important information.

If the sleeplessness is thought to be secondary to a sleep disorder, a PSG will be required. In fact, the patient may be requested to stay the next day and engage in a series of nap studies to determine the extent of her daytime sleepiness. In summary, insomnia symptoms rarely require PSG evaluation and daytime nap studies. When the sleep difficulty is considered to be more severe (in terms of behavior and health disturbance), the PSG and/or daytime nap studies will be required. The PSG is the gold standard method used to determine the correct diagnosis.

In comparison, actigraphy involves the use of a wrist monitor that records the intensity and frequency of movement. This is a wristwatch-like device that tracks movement in three dimensions. It has a small computer chip with a memory program that collects the data of the person's movements and compares that to an algorithm for sedentary and active movement. In this manner, reduced movement can be accurately categorized as either lying down quietly, presumably sleeping, and increased movement can be categorized as up and active, when a person is awake. Thus, the accuracy is in terms of nonactivity versus activity. The actigraph is worn constantly on the wrist and is only removed when bathing or anytime the person goes into water (i.e., going in a hot tub or swimming pool).

The findings from actigraph readings have been compared to all-night PSG studies, and results indicate the utility of actigraphs for determining sleep from wake periods. Actigraphy has limitations because it does not allow for calculation of sleep stages and does not discriminate between sleep and lying still while awake. Thus, inaccurate estimates of sleep parameters may result. Nevertheless, actigraphy is helpful in determining the level of daytime and nighttime activity, especially for individuals who complain of fragmented nocturnal sleep. It does provide a sleep fragmentation index (an algorithm that calculates the number of arousals and the duration that a person is awake). This fragmentation index provides the sleep specialist with valuable information about an individual's quality of sleep.

The actigraph is an expensive product that is used frequently in sleep research and in clinical care. You may want to discuss the specifics of its use with your sleep specialist because there are reimbursement codes that may be used. The memory on the actigraph varies with different manufacturers, although a two-week period is typical.

THE CLINICAL INTERVIEW

The questions asked during the clinical interview are intended to assist the sleep specialist in understanding, diagnosing, and formulating a treatment plan for your sleep disturbance. The questions are aimed at discovering what is troubling about your sleep and when you first noticed disturbed sleep. It is also very important to find out the reasons why an individual comes for evaluation and treatment when he does. It is logically presumed that the condition is severe enough, or sometimes the person is pressured sufficiently to seek care or practical issues present themselves that make treatment of the sleep disturbance possible (e.g., new medical benefits that reimburse for care). The sleep specialist interviewing the patient is seeking answers to questions of severity of sleep disturbance, timing of the sleep disturbance (beginning, middle, or end of the sleep period), frequency of the sleep difficulty (number of times per week), and duration of the symptom experience and daytime impairments (i.e., excessive daytime sleepiness).

Measurement of your sleep will begin with observation. Either directly or indirectly, the sleep specialist will observe the degree of fatigue and sleepiness that you are reporting. It is important to make the distinction between sleepiness and fatigue. Sleepiness relates to degree of alertness, whereas fatigue relates to energy levels. Additionally, you will be asked to respond to questions about your sleep. For instance, what are the main reasons that brought you to the sleep specialist? Your reasons may be varied and complicated; you will need to be as specific as possible. For instance, is your sleep complaint related to difficulty falling asleep, staying asleep, falling and staying asleep, or early-morning awakenings? Perhaps you feel that you have insufficient sleep, that you wake up feeling unrefreshed, or that your daily schedule (work, personal, or school) interferes with your sleep.

Three of the most valuable pieces of information that you can provide to your sleep specialist are when (month and date) your sleep problems first began, how the sleep difficulty first began (e.g., trouble falling asleep), and what events were occurring in your life during this time. This information allows the sleep specialist to determine how extensive the sleep disturbance is for you. It is likely that you will be asked to recall how your sleep has been in last two weeks or so. It would not be uncommon for you to be asked to keep track of your sleep with a sleep diary (also called a sleep log). A sleep diary is used to record a variety of information regarding your sleep. A sample sleep diary is illustrated in appendix 4.[2,3] For instance, you may be requested to document the time you went to bed, the amount of time it took you to fall asleep, the total number of awakenings, the total length of time awake during the night, any stressors you may have experienced, and if you took any medication or drank alcohol. The sleep log assists the sleep specialist in learning how disrupted your sleep is and what factors may be contributing to your disturbed sleep. The sleep log may also inquire about napping and the timing and duration of your napping. In general, it is a detailed description of what you do before sleep, during the night if you wake up, and your behaviors during the day. It is important that you report to the best of your ability all of the activities that you engage in, even though these behaviors may be counter to facilitating sleep.

You will also be asked about how your sleep affects your daytime functioning. Think in terms of how your sleep affects you cognitively, physically, psychologically, and behaviorally. For example, do you feel anxious and tense during the day or night? Do you worry in bed, and what are you worrying about? It is also quite common to inquire about your emotional functioning because it may be associated with your sleep disturbance. This inquiry may take the form of being asked extensive questions about your mood, particularly in terms of low mood, anxiety, and the degree of stress that you are experiencing. Be prepared to answer questions regarding your evening and nighttime habits as well as the activities that you engage in when your sleep is disrupted. Additionally, it is very common to inquire about your coping methods for handling stress, even if it involves actions that you are not pleased with, such as drinking alcohol or taking over-the-counter sleeping pills to facilitate sleep. Questions regarding the timing of when you sleep—specifically the regularity of this timing—will most likely be asked to determine your ease of falling and staying asleep.

Additionally, medical and physical questions will be asked during the interview. The sleep specialist may ask questions regarding leg movements, snoring, sleep-related breathing problems, dream activity, activity that may occur during sleep, and other factors that may disrupt sleep. You should also be prepared to list all the medications that you are currently taking to assist with falling asleep or staying awake, including recreational drugs and alternative herbal and vitamin therapies. Your sleep specialist may also inquire about types of food and whether you use alcohol, caffeine, or tobacco products. The timing of when you eat, drink alcohol or caffeine products, or use tobacco is important in understanding the potential external factors influencing your sleep. Last, it is likely that a complete physical may be conducted or ordered and medications or medical procedures will be ordered.

SELF-REPORT MEASURES

Self-report measures are generally always administered before the clinical visit takes place and provide the sleep specialist with important medical, behavioral, and psychological information. Sleep clinics generally administer standardized self-report measures. These measures take approximately 10 to 30 minutes to complete and inquire about stress level, medications, current health, sleep habits, medical history, mood functioning, signs, and symptoms necessitating the sleep appointment. Results are typically integrated into a report and include the interview data, physician interview remarks, any sleep testing (i.e., PSG, nap studies, actigraphy). With this report, you will have an idea of how your sleep difficulty is conceptualized and what the appropriate treatment recommendations are.

Sleep Notes

- All-night and daytime nap studies are commonly used to detect serious sleep disorders.
- Nonpharmaceutical treatments work.
- Counseling with a sleep specialist is generally short term.

Exercises

1. List three issues you want to discuss with your sleep specialist.

REFERENCES

1. Littner, M., Hirshkowitz, M., Kramer, M., Kapen, S., Anderson, W. M., Bailey, D. et al. (2003). Practice parameters for using polysomnography to evaluate insomnia: An update. *Sleep, 26,* 754–760.
2. Graci, G. M. (2005, September–October). Pathogenesis and management of cancer-related insomnia. *The Journal of Supportive Oncology, 3*(5), 349–359.
3. Mills, M., & Graci, G. (2004). Sleep disturbances. In M. Frogge (Ed.), *Cancer Symptom Management* (pp. 111–134). Sudbury, MA: Jones & Bartlett.

CHAPTER 5

Treatments for Sleep Disturbances

The treatments for sleep disturbances have been the focus of outstanding research investigations. Complex and rigorous scientific studies have yielded robust treatment outcomes. The rationale for utilizing various treatment interventions is based on the level of distress and behavioral discomfort experienced by patients.[1]

Sources of sleep disturbance in individuals are many, varied, and complex.[2] It is helpful to think of these sources in terms of predisposing, precipitating, and perpetuating factors.[1,2,3] Chronic insomnia has received the most attention from this conceptualization model (figure 5.1). The condition of chronic insomnia is conceptualized as starting from what are termed *predisposing factors*.[1,2] These factors are events or actions that significantly disturb one's sleep, such as anxious or tense feelings, and are sufficient factors leading to sleep disturbance (i.e., not being able to fall asleep and/or stay asleep). *Precipitating factors* are viewed as disturbing events that interrupt and worsen sleep. Examples of precipitating factors include experiencing a medical illness that causes extended wakefulness or being subjected to continued environmental disturbance such as loud music from a neighbor's apartment. Individuals then

Figure 5.1
Spielman and Glovinsky's model of sleep disturbance

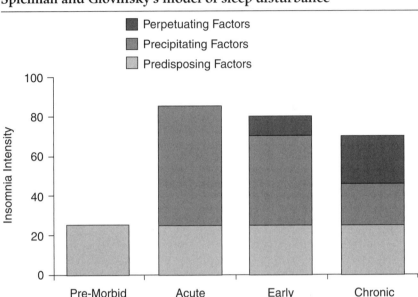

engage in behaviors to "fix" their sleep. These behaviors actually perpetuate the sleep disturbance instead of "fixing" sleep. For instance, individuals may decide to stay up really late by watching television to increase sleepiness. In this example, staying up late does not enhance sleep initiation; it succeeds only in making the individual more aroused instead of achieving a state of relaxation.

Two empirically validated sleep treatments are stimulus control and sleep restriction therapies; a brief description of each therapy and treatment rationale[2,4,5] are included in table 5.1. These approaches are quite effective with insomnia diagnoses and may even be applied to complaints of poor sleep that do not meet insomnia criteria. Occasional insomnia is common, and many factors may precipitate the sleep disturbance. Researchers have hypothesized an interrelationship between anxiety, depression, and insomnia[2] (figure 5.2).

Table 5.1
Description Rationale and Treatments for Sleep Disturbance

SLEEP THERAPY TREATMENTS:

STIMULUS CONTROL:

The overall goal of stimulus control is to train the patient, through a learning paradigm, to associate the bed with sleeping and sleeping with the bed. In addition, the patient learns to "set" his or her sleep/wake cycle.

SLEEP RESTRICTION:

Limiting time allowable in bed by creating a mild state of sleep deprivation

TREATMENT RATIONALE:
* alter dysfunctional beliefs and attitudes about sleep
* educate patients about healthier sleep practices
* alter dysfunctional beliefs and attitudes about sleep
* educate patients about healthier sleep practices

SLEEP RESTRICTION THERAPY

You are going to be asked to go on a so-called sleep diet. This type of intervention is formally called sleep restriction and represents one of the most effective means to regulate your sleep. By keeping track of your sleep with a sleep log, you will be able to convey to your sleep specialist the times during the day that you are sleeping (appendix 4). Be prepared to discuss events leading to wakefulness, the amount of time you lie awake, and the way you feel at bedtime and at wake time.

The logic behind the use of sleep restriction has been demonstrated in many research studies of sleep quality. Consolidating sleep to the actual time when one is sleeping (on a regular basis) provides the necessary cues to the brain that it is time to sleep.[3,6] It is also important that you associate the bed with sleeping and sleeping only. If you have associated your bedroom with reading, your sleep specialist will assist you in reformulating these thoughts

Figure 5.2
The interrelationship of anxiety, depression, and insomnia

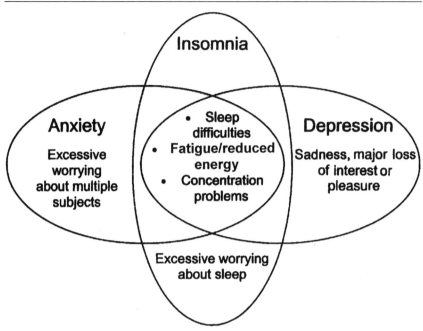

and feelings. A person may be able to fall asleep but perhaps wakes up and then cannot return to sleep until the body is ready for sleep. It is very common for individuals to lie awake in bed and focus on not sleeping and worrying about how this lack of sleep is going to affect them during the day.

Sleep restriction generally involves creating a mild state of sleep deprivation with the goal of increasing sleep pressure so that patients are able to consolidate their sleep. The overarching goal is to have the patient sleep continuously throughout the night. A general heuristic is that if you complain of difficulty falling asleep and report lying awake in bed for more than 30 minutes, your sleep specialist may restrict your bedtime to the actual time (on a consistent basis) that you report falling asleep. For instance, if a patient reports going to bed at 10:00 P.M. but does not fall asleep until midnight, it is appropriate to suggest going to bed at midnight.

STIMULUS CONTROL THERAPY

Wakefulness after sleep onset arising from an environmental trigger or behavioral factors has been studied extensively.[6] It seems that the longer an individual lies in bed ruminating or worrying about not sleeping can be the stimulus that produces the arousal or anxiety that is associated with either walking into your bedroom or getting into bed at night. Once the bedroom is associated with anxious feelings or sensation, the bed is no longer considered a safe haven. The wakefulness associated with worrying about not sleeping is sufficiently potent to cause not sleeping to be habit forming.

Stimulus control therapy is the treatment that involves breaking up these false bedroom associations or the conditioned arousal that we have taught ourselves to experience when we get into bed. If we learn to dread sleep, we can unlearn it through stimulus control treatment. The primary objective of stimulus control therapy is to train the patient, through a learning paradigm, to associate the bed with sleeping and sleeping with the bed. In addition, the patient learns to set their sleep-wake cycle. To achieve these goals, the following behaviors are suggested:

- Go to bed only when sleepy.
- Pursue only sleep in bed. No other activity except sexual activity is permitted; in other words, reading, eating, watching television, or completing homework is to be done not in bed but in another area of the home.
- Get out of bed if sleep does not come within 15 or 20 minutes of retiring at night, and engage in relaxing behavior, returning to bed only when sleepy (this may be repeated as often as needed throughout the night).

- Wake at the same time every day, regardless of the amount of sleep achieved during the night.
- Avoid daytime naps.

Essentially, the intervention entails having an individual get out of bed and go into another room if he is unable to sleep within 15 minutes and engaging in a *boring, non-mentally stimulating activity*. The key is that the activity has to be boring and non-mentally stimulating. The selection of a boring task is designed to neutralize one's dreadful thinking and, in effect, to promote relaxation that can elicit sleep. The boring task activity is done outside of the bedroom so as to break the link of the bedroom and sleeplessness. In numerous studies of this intervention, it has been consistently found to be one of the most effective.[6] Some individuals may have to repeat the procedure more than once a night in order to reduce or eliminate bodily tension and replace it with one of relaxation experienced from performing a boring task in the middle of the night.

HOW TO COMBINE SLEEP RESTRICTION AND STIMULUS CONTROL THERAPIES

After keeping a sleep log of your sleep habits for two weeks, you will want to review your bedtimes, wake times, and sleep times with your sleep specialist. The purpose of this review is to determine a consistent time when sleep is most likely to occur. For instance, if you are going to bed at 9:00 P.M. but lie in bed until 11:00 P.M. before falling asleep, your actual bedtime should be scheduled for 11:00 P.M.

This information derived from the sleep logs will assist your sleep specialist in calculating appropriate bedtimes and wake times. This intervention restricts the timing of sleep to whatever the sleep specialist determines is your appropriate sleep interval.

You are not to go to bed earlier than designated, and definitely do not to sleep later than your scheduled wake time. The use of an alarm clock ensures a regular wake time. At a physiological level, sleep restriction helps reset the brain to learn that you have new sleep and wake times. It is considered to be an effective technique because it also consolidates a person's sleep. Go to bed only when sleepy. Make adjustments to your new schedule. The relationship between all of these suggestions is illustrated in figure 5.3.[1] We cannot overemphasize the importance of establishing prebedtime rituals to promote relaxation, avoiding daytime naps, and establishing regular sleep habits. These behaviors facilitate relaxation, thereby promoting the onset and maintenance of sleep.

Figure 5.3
Conceptualization of sleep-scheduling treatments

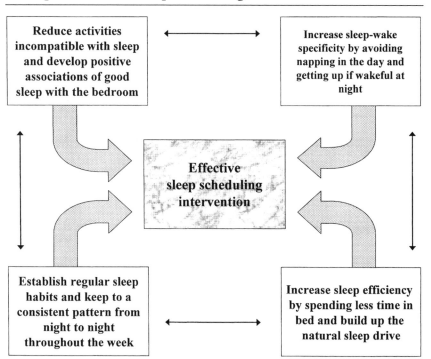

Sleep Notes

- Sleep treatments are carefully planned to ensure effectiveness.
- Necessary paperwork, such as sleep logging and some self-report measures, helps plan for where changes in sleep must be made.
- Reasonable modifications are effective in adjusting your sleep.

Exercises

1. What are your boring tasks that you will do when you have difficulty either falling asleep or have an awakening lasting more than 15 minutes?
2. How is your sleep going to be restructured? Describe how you will consolidate your bed and wake times and how they will change over the next three to four weeks.

REFERENCES

1. Morin, C. M., & Espie, C. A. (Eds.). (2003). *Insomnia: A clinical guide to assessment and treatment.* New York: Kluwer Academic/Plenum.
2. Graci, G. (2005, September–October). Pathogenesis and management of cancer-related insomnia. *The Journal of Supportive Oncology, 3*(5), 349–359.
3. Spielman, A. J., & Glovinsky, P. (1991). The varied nature of insomnia. In P. J. Hauri (Ed.), *Case Studies of Insomnia.* New York: Springer. (pp. 1–15).
4. Graci, G., & Sexton-Radek, K. (2005). Treating sleep disorders using cognitive behavioral therapy and hypnosis. In R. A. Chapman (Ed.), *The clinical use of hypnosis in cognitive behavior therapy: A practitioner's casebook* (p. 348). New York: Springer.
5. Mills, M., & Graci, G. (2004). Sleep disturbances. In M. Frogge (Ed.), *Cancer symptom management* (pp. 111–134). Sudbury, MA: Jones & Bartlett.
6. Perlis, M. L., & Lichstein, K. L. (2003). *Treating sleep disorders: Principles and practice of behavioral sleep medicine.* New York: Wiley.

CHAPTER 6

Change Your Mind about Your Sleep

Many individuals who have difficulty sleeping begin to worry about their lack of sleep and the nightly struggle to achieve restful sleep. They may ruminate more about their sleep patterns than the current stressors they are experiencing. This excessive thinking leads to developing thoughts that only amplify the problem. For instance, sleep difficulties may be seen as a potential contributor to ongoing problems. You may become concerned, as one recent patient did, that lack of sleep will result in poor job performance, which will result inevitably in termination from employment and loss of the family's resources that will preclude his children (ages 5 and 12) from going to college and achieving successful careers. You may ask, "How do I stop this excessive thinking from happening?" If you are working with a sleep specialist, you may be challenged on the truth or validity of these statements and encouraged to produce alternative thoughts. Then you may be encouraged to compare the truth of your worried thoughts to the alternatives.

The following discussion illustrates how a sleep specialist can help you change your mind about sleep. Two main factors are pivotal in changing your sleep: thinking (what are you thoughts) and behaving (things you do that affect sleep) factors. The assumption is that thoughts influence behaviors.[1,2] Individuals experiencing disturbed sleep commonly focus much of their attention on the disturbance and how it impacts their lives.

This thinking or focused attention becomes problematic when we create faulty assumptions about sleep, including how we sleep and what helps our sleep. As a result of these faulty beliefs, inappropriate or compulsive behaviors are established. For example, excessively thinking about why we are not falling asleep somehow will solve our problem of not sleeping. The excessive cognitive activity is actually a mentally stimulating activity that does not promote relaxation, however; instead it creates a heightened state of arousal that is not conducive to sleep. Faulty beliefs or behaviors can also materialize from having insufficient knowledge or understanding about sleep. This lack of knowledge, or sleep myths, occurs because television and other media sources can misrepresent or generalize sleep facts that may or may not apply to your sleep. For example, the media often reports that individuals need eight hours of sleep in order to feel rested and function at optimal levels. Some individuals, however, may require eight hours of sleep, whereas others may require either five hours (short sleepers) or ten hours (long sleepers) to feel refreshed and rested. A short sleeper by nature (less than six hours) generally will not be able to consistently achieve eight hours of sleep per night. Biologically, these individuals are not wired for eight hours of sleep, and it is not in their best interest to try to calculate when they should go to bed in order to get eight hours of sleep. The average adult sleep period, taking into account different age groups, is approximately seven hours and 15 minutes.[3] Given this finding, it is not surprising that individuals may inappropriately worry or become anxious that they

Figure 6.1
Potential factors contributing to sleep disturbance

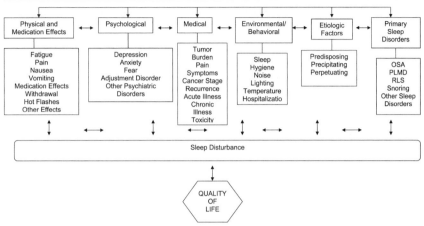

are not achieving the so-called required eight hours of sleep per night.

Are faulty beliefs or behaviors regarding sleep the only factors that can disturb sleep? Unfortunately, many other factors can fragment or shorten sleep (figure 6.1).[3] The most common factors include, but are not limited to, emotional upset (e.g., worrying, anxiety), pain, psychological syndromes, and/or medical disorders.[4] Many individuals worry or focus their attention on unresolved or problematic issues, specifically at night. Nighttime is generally the one time when we have alone or down time. Unfortunately, we often do not make the time for processing thoughts, events, or feelings that we may be experiencing earlier in the day. As a result of this neglect, sleep is shortened because nighttime now takes on a new meaning: Our minds become active and our bodies tense, and these events intrude on our sleep.

The sleep specialist can assist you in identifying your problematic thinking or discovering the behaviors that you engage in that may disturb sleep. Problematic thinking is addressed by exploring your feelings about sleep and how your sleep affects you. This process is accomplished in a step-by-step manner of introducing new, alternative beliefs or behaviors to replace problematic ones. For example, questions may include, "What was on your mind when you could not sleep?" Patient responses to questions such as this one will yield important information in assisting your sleep specialist in restoring your sleep.

Challenging faulty thoughts or beliefs about sleep may seem overwhelming, but the purpose is to change these thoughts or beliefs to more realistic ones—something that *can* be accomplished. The overarching goal is to end your sleep struggles by providing you with techniques and behaviors that will help you sleep. These techniques and behaviors, when practiced correctly, help build confidence that you can sleep, you really can!

How do I make the change, you may ask? You can achieve change either by yourself or with your sleep specialist. An adaptation of the theoretical model of change to this issue of sleep is presented in figure 6.2. This model of change is important in understanding the necessary changes you will have to make to restore and improve your sleep. The model has five steps: precontemplation, contemplation, preparation, action, and maintenance. Each of these steps will be discussed in detail.

In precontemplation, an individual has limited information about the problem (sleep disturbance) or lacks insight about the sleep disturbance, resulting in inadequate attention and motivation for change. The next stage, contemplation, relates to an individual's willingness to learn about sleep disturbance. For example, if you are reading this book to help you understand and solve your sleep struggles, then you are in the contemplation stage of change. You are learning about sleep so that you can apply this knowledge to solve your sleep difficulties. The preparation phase involves implementing or experimenting with behavioral changes. For instance, the preparation phase may include tracking

Figure 6.2
The five stages of change required to solve your sleep struggles

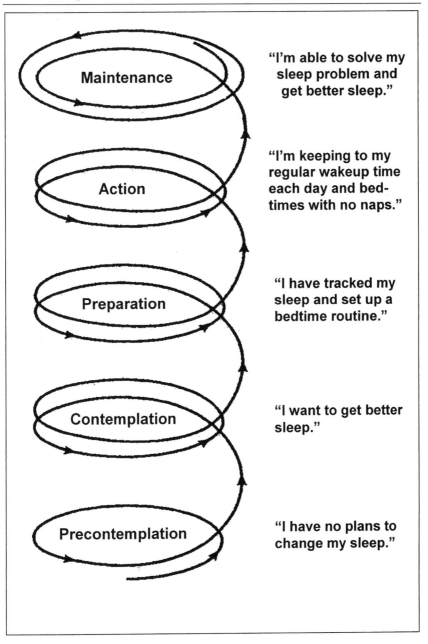

your sleep by recording it in a sleep diary or journal format. The tracking is necessary for implementing a sleep schedule that is consistent with the time when you are sleepiest at night. Sleep scheduling not only conditions your body to sleep at the appropriate time (when you are most sleepy) but also provides your body with the appropriate number of hours that your body naturally requires. Changing your timing of sleep is the first change made in the preparation phase because it is the most effective. The next stage, action, is continuation of the preparation stage in that an individual becomes more active in making or implementing behavioral changes. This increase in implementing behavioral changes (activity) strengthens an individual's commitment and probability for success. In this stage, it is important to ensure that the behavioral changes can be easily accomplished. Let us return to our preparation stage example. After an individual has tracked her sleep and established a regular sleep schedule, introducing behaviors and factors that help her sleep better is appropriate. These factors are termed *sleep hygiene behaviors*.[5,6,7] This term was coined years ago when implementation of good health behaviors were called *hygiene*.

Maintenance is the final stage of change, and it involves developing a long-term plan to sustain the changes that have been accomplished. There is a sense of competence and success that occurs in the maintenance stage. The individual no longer struggles with sleep, rather she has developed the belief (through actions/behaviors) that she is capable of maintaining the behaviors necessary for good sleep. Minor setbacks are addressed by implementing contingency plans to assist with readjusting behaviors to achieve good and refreshing sleep. An example of a contingency plan would include developing a plan for readjusting one's sleep routine that may have been altered by vacation, illness, and/or personal circumstances.

Sleep Notes

- Your thinking influences your behavior, including your sleep.

Exercises

1. What are some of your beliefs about why you struggle with sleep?
2. What are some of the things you do (behaviors) that influence your sleep?

REFERENCES

1. Van Egeren, L., Haynes, S. N., Franzen, M., & Hamilton, J. (1983). Pre-sleep cognitions and attributions in sleep-onset insomnia. *Journal of Behavioral Medicine, 6*(2), 217–232.
2. Harvey, A. G. (2002). A cognitive model of insomnia. *Behavior Research and Therapy, 40*(8), 869–893.
3. Kryger, M. H., Roth, T. & Dement. W. C. (2005). *Principles and practice of sleep medicine.* (4th ed.). Philadelphia: Saunders.
4. Graci, G. (2005, September–October). Pathogenesis and management of cancer-related insomnia. *The Journal of Supportive Oncology, 3*(5), 349–359.
5. Prochaska, J. O., Norcross, J. C., & DiClemente, C. C. (1994). *Systems of psychotherapy: A transtheoretical analysis.* New York: Brooks Cole.
6. Hauri, P. J. (2001). Insomnia. In *National sleep medicine course.* Leesburg, VA: American Academy of Sleep Medicine.
7. Hauri, P. (1989). The cognitive-behavioral treatment of insomnia. In A. Baum (Ed.), *Eating, sleeping and sex: Perspectives in behavioral medicine* (pp. 181–194). Hillsdale, NJ: Erlbaum.

CHAPTER 7

Alternative Treatments for Sleep

The interest in alternative care began in 1999 when several foundations (e.g., the National Institutes of Health Center for Complimentary and Alternative Medicine and Centers for Disease Control and Prevention) began researching and exploring clinical use of alternative medicine.[1] In recent years, it has become increasingly popular and more accepting for health care centers to provide some form of alternative medicine. These alternative medicine techniques traditionally include hypnosis, meditation, massage therapy, exercise, and biofeedback.

Although alternative medicine approaches have not received the scientific support that behavioral techniques have received for improving sleep, they are very popular and widely used (e.g., self-help magazines, talk shows, and radio programs). These media outlets discuss the benefits of alternative medicine approaches to improving sleep functioning. For example, much emphasis has been placed on the utilization of nutrition, exercise, and aromatherapy to improve sleep.

Nutrition with regard to sleep entails the type and timing of meals.[1,2,3] People who engage in regular eating patterns are generally observed to have good sleep.[1] In contrast, sleep-deprived individuals are more likely to ingest high-calorie foods (i.e., sugars) and greater quantities of food because of the belief that food will replenish energy deficits. It is recommended that individuals avoid ingestion of heavy meals before bedtime (they induce digestion, which requires metabolic energy and is alerting).

You may ask, "Are there any foods that promote sleep?" There are many folktales about milk or other foods leading to good sleep. These findings have not been substantiated in research settings; however, milk and turkey contain a chemical that is involved in generating a sleep-inducing agent in the brain. More research is needed in this area to determine the relationship between these foods and this neurological sleep-inducing agent.

Grocery stores and homeopathic vendors sell a plethora of herbal and aromatherapy remedies. More popular sleep-inducing herbal and aroma agents include valerian, hops, chamomile, lavender, passion flower, and lemon balm aromas.[1,3] Researches have not been able to determine the appropriate amount of these agents needed to induce sleep. Additionally, administration, in terms of timing (when to take them), and the mechanism of action of these agents are unknown. Due to an unknown safety profile, we do not recommend taking any of these agents in large quantities.

The majority of Americans have difficulty quieting their minds at night. It is becoming ever more popular to problem solve at bedtime. We know that problem solving is a mentally stimulating activity and interferes with sleep facilitation. Several alternative interventions are efficacious in assisting individuals to deploy their attention away from problem solving or worrying. These interventions include relaxation training, guided imagery, yoga, and meditation.

Relaxation training assists an individual with easing and quieting both mind and body. It involves using a series of directive statements that suggest releasing tension from various areas of the body (arms, legs, fingers, toes, head, etc.).[4,5] Measured changes in heart rate, muscle tone, blood pressure, and reductions in pain medication use are frequently observed in individuals participating in treatment frequently.[4] Relaxation has been found to be effective for a number of physical and psychological disorders, including high blood pressure, epilepsy, pain, anxiety, and depression, and in the treatment of somatized tension associated with insomnia.[1]

Relaxation has been broadened to include promoting the relaxation response by using multiple sensory modalities (thinking of relaxing scenes in guided imagery exercises), listening to relaxing sounds or music, and using temperature control (usually slight heat) to induce relaxation. Many companies specializing in self-help products have scripted tapes with sound, music, and vocal accompaniment to promote at-home relaxation. You may find it helpful to sample a few tapes before buying them to determine which type of relaxation tape or compact disc is appropriate for you. We have included two sample relaxation scripts for your use (appendix 8).[6]

Furthermore, meditation and yoga approaches have received a lot attention in the last several years. Meditation and yoga also require some directed instruction and practice to master the techniques. Similar to relaxation training, meditation and yoga can induce a relaxation response, but by a different pathway. The history of meditation and yoga is rich with philosophical, spiritual, and mythical proponents to its use and practice. Self-study and practice are essential. The practice of meditation and yoga entails the use of controlling your body through slowed breathing and using chanting to develop this slow rhythm to breathing and incorporating muscle relaxation by performing different stretches and postures. To gain the benefits of these techniques, an individual must refocus her thoughts, emotions, and physical responses while engaging in the various positions that promote relaxation and mental and physical balance. Continued practice makes this a skill that can be invoked when needed. It is important to note that yoga and meditation both require directed instruction.

In addition to yoga and meditation, exercise is also helpful to sleep. Exercise (on a consistent basis and done four to six hours before bedtime) not only improves sleep but also promotes deep sleep.[3] Furthermore, individuals who exercise regularly have been found to report lower incidences of mood disturbance (anxiety and depression) and sleep problems.[7] The positive benefits of exercise do not stop here. In addition to the healthy effects exercise has been found to have on the heart, lungs, blood pressure, and muscle mass, exercise also increases feelings of control, independence, and self-esteem and improves sleep efficiency (time spent in bed/time spent asleep) and ratings of sleep quality (excellent, good, fair, poor sleep).

We also know that overweight individuals tend to report more health problems, including poor sleep. One of the sleep problems associated with obesity or weight gain is an increased risk of obstructive sleep apnea. Patients diagnosed with sleep apnea are instructed to reduce their weight because excess fat surrounding the neck and throat areas increases the chance that the airway will become obstructed during sleep, causing apnea (periods when breathing stops) to occur. Weight gain also increases snoring. Reduction in body mass decreases the burden on the heart and lungs. Sleep difficulties can worsen a weight problem. Individuals with insomnia sometimes eat in their wakeful hours of the night and/or overeat during the day in hopes that food will give them energy. As one can see, exercise is both healthy for the body and a good sleep agent.

Last, a discussion on implementation of good or adaptive sleep hygiene behaviors is essential in helping you achieve sleep. Sleep hygiene refers to the organization of activities (e.g., presleep behaviors) that promote sleep and minimize sleep disturbance. Typically, it incorporates the following behaviors:

- Reduce the intake of nicotine, caffeine, and other stimulants.
- Avoid stimulants (if taken) in the afternoon or evening.
- Avoid alcohol near bedtime.
- Keep a regular daytime schedule for work, rest, meals, treatment, exercise, and other daily activities.
- Perform strenuous exercises early in the day rather than in the late afternoon or evening.

Good sleep hygiene means modifying one's environment and lifestyle.[3,8] The National Sleep Foundation provides a more comprehensive list of healthy sleep tips (table 7.1). Insomnia complaints can often be corrected by implementing these proper sleep hygiene behaviors. For instance, some individuals are reluctant to avoid napping during the day, or they will unintentionally fall asleep during the day. This unintentional sleep is often a major contributor to the onset and maintenance of insomnia. The goal is to educate the patient so that he can eliminate behaviors that lead to sleep disturbance. A sleep specialist can teach you how to apply both lifestyle and bedroom factors that promote sleep (figure 7.1).

Table 7.1
Sleep Tips Promoting a Healthy Sleep Style

Keep a regular sleep schedule. Our sleep-wake cycles are regulated by a "circadian clock" in our brain and the body's need to balance sleep and wake times. It is beneficial to go to bed and get up at the same time each night to allow your body to get in sync with this natural pattern. Keeping a regular bed and wake-time, even on the weekends when there is the temptation to "sleep-in," will make it easier for you to fall asleep and maintain sleep quality throughout the week.

Avoid caffeine. Caffeine is a stimulant, which means it can keep you awake. Caffeinated products, such as coffee, tea, cola and chocolate, remain in the body on average from 3 to 5 hours, but they can affect some people up to 12 hours later. Consuming caffeine in the afternoon or evening can disrupt sleep, so it is important to monitor your caffeine intake late in the afternoon. Even if you do not think that caffeine affects you, it may be disrupting your sleep. Avoiding caffeine within 6 hours of going to bed can help improve sleep quality.

Avoid nicotine. Nicotine is also a stimulant. Smoking before bed makes it more difficult to fall asleep. When smokers go to sleep, they experience withdrawal from nicotine, which also causes problems falling asleep or waking in the morning. Nicotine can also cause nightmares. Difficulty sleeping is just one more reason to quit smoking.

Avoid alcohol. Although many people think of alcohol as a sleep aid because of its sedating effect, it causes more sleep disruptions throughout the night. Consuming alcohol before bedtime usually helps people to relax and fall asleep, but can lead to a night of disturbed sleep.

(Continued)

Table 7.1 (continued)

Don't eat or drink too much close to bedtime. Eating or drinking too much may make you less comfortable when settling down for bed. It is best to avoid a heavy meal too close to bedtime. Also, spicy foods may cause heartburn, which leads to difficulty falling asleep and discomfort during the night. Try to restrict fluids close to bedtime to prevent nighttime awakenings to go to the bathroom. On the other hand, going to bed hungry may also make it more difficult to sleep. A light snack is often best before bed and may help you sleep better.

Exercise at the right time promotes sleep. In general, exercise makes it easier to fall asleep and contributes to sounder sleep. However, exercising right before going to bed will make falling and staying asleep more difficult. In addition to making us more alert, body temperature rises during exercise, and takes about six hours to begin to drop. A cooler body temperature signals the body that it is time to sleep. Exercise, but do so at least three hours before bedtime. Late afternoon exercise will help you fall asleep at night.

Use relaxing bedtime rituals. A relaxing, routine activity right before bedtime will make it easier to fall asleep. Avoid stimulating activities like working and exercise that can make it more difficult to fall asleep. Try an activity that is relaxing such as taking a hot bath, reading or listening to music. If you are unable to avoid tension and stress, it may be helpful to learn relaxation techniques from a trained professional.

Create a sleep-promoting environment. Most people sleep best in an environment that is cool, quiet and dark. Check your room for noise or other distractions, including a bed partner's sleep disruptions or an environment that is too bright, too dry or humid, or too hot or cold. Make sure your mattress is comfortable and supportive for you and your bedpartner.

IF YOU HAVE DIFFICULTY SLEEPING...

Associate your bed with sleep and sex only. Use your bed only for sleep and sex to strengthen the psychological association between bed and sleep. Follow a regular wake-up schedule.

Avoid watching the clock. If you associate a particular activity or item with anxiety about sleeping, omit it from your bedtime routine. For example, if looking at a bedroom clock makes you anxious about how much time you have before you must get up, move the clock out of sight. Do not engage in activities that cause anxiety and prevent you from sleeping.

Limit sleep time in bed. If you have difficulty sleeping, go to bed only when you are tired. If you do not fall asleep within 15 minutes, it is best to get out

Table 7.1 (continued)

of bed and do another relaxing activity until you feel sleepy again. Repeat if necessary. If worrying about something you need to do prevents you from sleeping, it is sometimes helpful to jot down notes in a "to do" book. Nap during the day only when needed and plan on napping just 20-30 minutes.

Use a sleep diary and talk to your doctor. Try these tips and record your sleep and sleep-related activities in a sleep diary. If problems continue, discuss the sleep diary with your doctor. There may be an underlying cause for your sleep problem, and you will want to be properly diagnosed. Your doctor will help treat the problem or may refer you to a sleep specialist.

Source: National Sleep Foundation.

Figure 7.1
Lifestyle and bedroom factors: a complete list of sleep hygiene factors

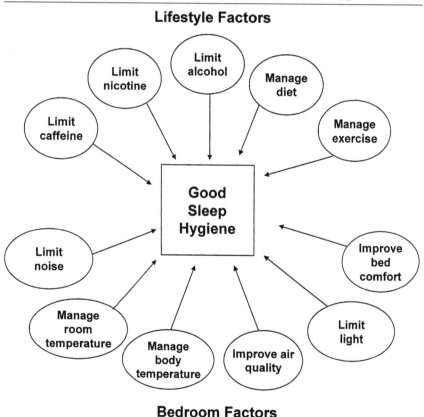

Sleep Notes

- Despite substantial scientific evidence for some approaches, alternative interventions are very popular.
- Monitor food intake sensibly.
- Relaxation, meditation, and yoga training are useful techniques to induce mental and physical relaxation with an added benefit of quieting the mind.
- Exercise is not only good for you, it also deepens sleep.
- Sleep hygiene behaviors are behaviors that help facilitate sleep.

Exercises

1. Consider the following activities and add additional ones that you would like to consider participating in to promote mental and physical relaxation. Share this list with your sleep specialist at your next appointment.

   Nutrition/food intake

   Relaxation practice

   Meditation or yoga class

   Purchasing guided imagery or relaxation audiotapes or compact discs

   Exercise class or exercise on your own

   Sleep hygiene

2. List at least three things that you do that potentially could disrupt your sleep.

3. Can you replace these three things with more adaptive or alternative behaviors? What are these alternative behaviors?

REFERENCES

1. Freeman, L. W, & Lawlis, G. F. (2001). *Mosby's complimentary and alternative medicine: A research-based approach*. St. Louis, MO: Mosby Harcourt Health Sciences.

2. Fisher, C. S. (1982). *To dwell among friends: Personal networks in town and city*. Chicago: University of Chicago Press.

3. Dement, W. C., & Vaughn, C. (1999). *The promise of sleep*. New York: Random House.

4. Jacobson, F. (1938). *Progressive relaxation* (2nd ed.). Chicago: University of Chicago Press.

5. Benson, H., Greenwood, M. M., & Klenchuk, H. (1976). The relaxation response: Psychophysiological aspects and clinical applications. *International Journal of Psychiatry Medicine, 6*(1/2), 87.

6. Graci, G., & Sexton-Radek, K. (2005). Treating sleep disorders using cognitive behavioral therapy and hypnosis. In R. A. Chapman (Ed.), *The clinical use of hypnosis in cognitive behavior therapy: A practitioner's casebook* (pp. 295-323). New York: Springer.

7. Mock, V., Dow, K. H., Meares, C. J., Grimm, P. M., Dienemann, J. A., Haisfield-Wolfe, M. E., et al. (1997). Effects of exercise on fatigue, physical functioning, and emotional distress during radiation therapy for breast cancer. *Oncology Nursing Forum, 24,* 991–1000.

8. Stevenson, C., & Ernst, E. (2000). Valerian for insomnia: A systematic review of randomized clinical trials. *Sleep Medicine, 1,* 91–99.

Chapter 8

Follow-Up Care

As you begin reading this chapter, please remind yourself about what you have learned about sleep. Hopefully, this information will assist you in disarming the strong urge to struggle with sleep. You can determine what your body's sleep need is, sleep style, and ways to adjust your lifestyle to achieve good, restorative sleep. Keep in mind that sleep is a natural cycle with which you do not need to struggle but just give way to.[1,2]

Individuals who not only contemplate but also act on the decision to make sleep changes will experience better sleep.[2] Our experience has shown that patients in treatment with a sleep specialist show significant sleep changes. The strongest area of measured change was ratings of sleep quality followed by a reduction in time spent falling asleep and in the number of awakenings.[1,3] The last area of change was a reduction in the amount of time spent awake after waking up in the middle of the night.

We have provided you with information on how to deactivate the tension (all of those stressors!) so many of us experience at night. This deactivation allows you to embrace sleep and let go of any stressful thoughts or problems for the night. Nighttime, specifically bedtime, is for sleeping and allowing the body to restore itself, both physically and emotionally. Bedtime is not for worrying or problem solving.

Our book is designed to be an accompaniment to helping you solve your sleep struggles, especially if you are working with a sleep specialist. The aim is to educate you about sleep and empower you with the knowledge of why sleep can be disturbed and ways to solve the struggles. We have included in the appendixes of this book some additional resources that you may find helpful. These additional resources were written for sleep professionals and none were written for the person struggling with sleep who is contemplating going to a sleep specialist or has already begun treatment with a specialist. We know this information will help you solve your sleep troubles.

REFERENCES

1. Perlis, M. L., Jungquist, C., Smith, M. T., & Posner, D. (2005). *Cognitive behavioral treatment of insomnia: A session by session guide.* New York: Springer.
2. Harvey, A. G., & Payne, S. (2002). The management of unwanted pre-sleep thoughts in insomnia: Distraction with imagery versus general distraction. *Behavioral Research and Therapy, 40,* 267–277.
3. Perlis, M. L., & Lichstein, K. L. (2003). *Treating sleep disorders: Principles and practice of behavior medicine.* New York: Wiley.

Section Two
Common Sleep Battles

COMMON BATTLES

If you are reading this chapter, it is highly likely that your sleep is disturbed and you are searching for ways to battle this disturbance. Section one informed you of the common struggles and treatments related to sleep disorders, and this section will assist you even further in solving your sleep disturbance. If you use all of the principles discussed, you will have no more sleepless nights.

Sleep specialists use many different approaches to identify and treat sleep disturbance. These approaches include first identifying the nature of the sleep disturbance. Once the signs and symptoms of this difficulty are known, interventions focused on the pertinent issues can be implemented. Knowledge about signs and symptoms also include finding out when the sleep disturbance began. Was there anything occurring during this time that may have been stressful? Keep in mind that happy events can also be stressful. For example, we once had a patient who denied experiencing anything stressful during the time that her sleep disturbance began. After further investigation, she recalled that she was planning her wedding but did not consider this event stressful! Once we have the information that identifies the nature of the sleep disturbance, effective treatments can be implemented to alleviate the sleep disturbance.[1]

Many common day-to-day occurrences or situations can disturb sleep. Based on our clinical findings from working with patients reporting sleep disturbance, we feel some frequently experienced patterns of sleep disturbance stem from lifestyle factors. This section highlights some of these common lifestyle factors that affect sleep. Identification of these lifestyle factors and treatment suggestions are provided in order to help you resolve your sleep disturbance and assist you in working more effectively with a sleep specialist.

COLLEGE STUDENTS AND THEIR SLEEPINESS

Daytime sleepiness is a frequent sign of sleep deprivation or, as we like to label it, "depriving your mind, body, and spirit" of a necessary component to life: sleep. The major downside to sleep deprivation is that it affects our safety and can jeopardize our overall physical and emotional well-being. Sleep deprivation is commonly associated with motor vehicle accidents, work accidents, athletic injury, low productivity, and interference with daily activities. In a large-scale study, researchers identified the relationship between daytime sleepiness and short sleep duration, somatic distress, and insomnia symptoms in young adults.[2] Upon further questioning in interviews, researchers reported that young adults with excessive daytime sleepiness also reported trouble falling asleep, awakening during nighttime sleep, and nocturnal anxiety. In general, a bad night of sleep is linked to daytime sleepiness.

Factors such as communal living, altered lifestyle schedule (e.g., adaptation to residence hall and college life from home life), along with increased academic responsibility trouble young adults' sleep. Interestingly, a gender gap has been found on this issue, with women reporting more excessive daytime sleepiness than men.[3]

Thus quality of life is impaired for these young people on the threshold of beginning their lives as autonomous individuals.

Researchers commonly emphasize the public health risks associated with sleep deprivation, but attention should be given to our young adult population who often drive while sleepy. Despite feeling fatigue and sleepiness, college students, in one study, were found to be *more* likely to take risks while driving.[2] The average age for motor vehicle accidents is 25 years old;[4] however, more than 55 percent of these accidents occur at a median age of 20 years.[4] In fact, reports indicate the two highest peaks in motor vehicle accidents occur between ages 18 and 20 years and older than 56 years. Dozing due to sleepiness was the most common cause of these motor vehicle accidents. Young students were identified as the age group most at risk. The rate of accidents increases as the distance (in miles) from home or campus increases. Researchers identified specific incidents experienced by sleepy young adult drivers who were involved in motor vehicle accidents.[2] The most severe incident was considered to be momentarily falling asleep at the wheel, followed by completely falling asleep at the wheel with no consequence to the cars, changing lanes or moving to the shoulder, or having the automobile leave the road entirely. Last, youngest students (per class rank) were found to be at greatest risk.

Young adult females report more daily sleepiness, poor nighttime sleep, and not feeling refreshed in the morning than do young adult males[5] In general, most self-report studies (i.e., studies that use questionnaires to gain scientific information) indicate that females sleep less than men in terms of total nighttime sleep.[5] This sleep habit places females at a major disadvantage in being vulnerable to experiencing other sleep-related behaviors (i.e., poor sleep hygiene behaviors) and/or other sleep-related disorders (e.g., psychophysiological insomnia, hypnotic dependent sleep disorder).

Furthermore, sleep habits of young adults and older adults were found to be similar.[6] The major difference found, however, was that poor sleep factors predicted poor sleep in older adults. Interestingly, the researchers were unable to determine what may contribute to daytime sleepiness and poor nighttime sleep of young adults complaining of sleep disturbance. Additionally, these researchers also found that young adults reported lower levels of sleepiness compared to an older adult population. It may be the case that reporting and identifying daytime sleepiness is more complicated than we thought.

If time is available, young adults are more likely to resolve sleepiness by napping. Approximately 76 percent of young adults take naps,[7] indicating that this population naps more frequently with so-called power naps lasting, on average, 17.1 minutes. Power napping seems to be a self-corrective measure to remedy the variable sleep patterns that are typical of young adults.

Like health behaviors, sleep behaviors also affect academic performance. The grade point average is used to measure academic performance, and many student behaviors can influence this grade point average. For instance, sleep deprivation has a negative influence on performance, awareness, problem solving, and so forth. Additionally, health habits combined with good sleep habits, such as engaging in proper nutrition, exercise, utilizing social support systems, and using time and stress management techniques, should be a daily staple in everyone's life, not just students' lives. The next section provides more detailed information on how to employ these healthy habits into your life and ways to avoid sleepiness.

WAYS TO AVOID SLEEPINESS

NUTRITION

Eat breakfast. Although little research has focused on college students' academic performance and nutrition, we know this works for elementary-level children,[7] as a necessary component to fuel up their brains and jump-start their metabolism for the day. Furthermore, engaging in proper nutrition not only at breakfast but also throughout the day will keep you feeling more alert and less sleepy.

EMOTIONAL BALANCE

Explore and commit to some type of stress management practice to buffer the effects of depression and anxiety. Music, exercise, relaxation techniques (e.g., yoga, deep breathing, and guided imagery), and scheduled leisure activities are just a few type of activities that are effective in altering mood.

SOCIAL SUPPORT

Find who makes up your social support system. It may not necessarily be people you know or are close to. For example, it can be spiritual, intellectual, or social companionship. Once you identify who and what makes up your social support system, be sure to maintain it.

TIME MANAGEMENT

Daytimers' survey of young adults revealed that 67 percent work at least 10 hours per week and 47 percent use a personal planner to track their appointments and activities.[8] Increased focus on utilizing personal planners, whether these planners are paper or electronic devices, may help in this area. Daytimers' survey also reported that young adults feel constantly rushed, and those who used time management devices accomplished 76 percent of what they planned.

A REGULAR SLEEP SCHEDULE

Maintain a regular bedtime and wake time all seven days of the week. Research in this area has identified those students who went

to bed later during the weekend and awakened later the corresponding day compared to their weekday bedtimes experienced decreased
ability to recall complex material learned in class earlier that week.[9]

REFERENCES

1. Graci, G. & Sexton-Radek, K. (2006). Treating sleep disorders using
   cognitive behavioral therapy and hypnosis. In R. A. Chapman (Ed.)
   *The Clinical Use of Hypnosis in Cognitive Behavioral Therapy: A practioner's
   casebook.*, (pp. 295–323). New York: Springer Publishing
2. Lindsay, G. A., & Hanks, W. A. (1999). Descriptive epidemiology of
   dozing and driving in a college student population. *Journal of American
   College Health, 47*(4), 157–162.
3. Sexton-Radek, K. (2004). *Sleep quality in young adults.* New York: Edwin
   Mellon Press.
4. Hasler, G., Buysse, D. J., Ganna, A., Ajdacic, V., Eich, D., Rossler, W.,
   et al. (2005). Excessive daytime sleepiness in young adults: A 20-year
   prospective community study. *Journal of Clinical Psychiatry, 66*(4), 521–
   529.
5. Lindberg, E., Janson, C., Gislason, T., Bjornsson, E., Hetta, J., &
   Boman, G. (1997). Sleep disturbances in a young adult population:
   Can gender differences be explained by difference in psychological
   status? *Sleep, 20*(6), 381–387.
6. Pilcher, J. J., Schoeling, S. E., & Prosansky, C. M. (2000). Self-report
   sleep habits as predictors of subjective sleepiness. *Behavioral Medicine,
   25*(4), 161–169.
7. Pilcher, J. J., Michalowski, K. R., & Carrigan, R. D. (2001). The prevalence of daytime napping and its relationship to nighttime sleep. *Behavior Medicine, 27*, 71–76.
8. Daytimer (2007). High school student's and their time. Retrieved June 6,
   2007, from http://www.daytimer.com/timemanagementresources.
9. Dotto, I. (1996). Sleep stages, memory and learning. *Canadian Medical
   Association Journal, 154*(8), 1193–1196.

WHAT YOU CAN DO TO ENSURE HEALTHY SLEEP HABITS

1. Work with your sleep specialist and perhaps with members or faculty of your college community on your course schedule. For example, if you are not a morning person, do not schedule classes during this time if you can avoid it.
2. Do what you can to schedule good, regular sleep. Research in this area has established the association between an adequate sleep period with the anticipated number of REM periods as necessary for learning.[1,2,3,4] It is hypothesized that memory processing takes place during REM as measured by increased amounts of REM following learning tasks in research participants.
3. Establish a regular schedule by making your study/activity/everything else schedule on a daily basis. Schedule no more than two-hour study periods with breaks in between in a quiet place. Determine when assignments are due, figure out what needs to be done to accomplish assignments, and distribute those study actions over a period of time. Check your notes with the textbook and/or professor, rewrite your notes, and then consolidate these notes to concepts in a map format for review.
4. See a sleep specialist if your sleep disturbance and daytime sleepiness extends beyond a week and is not due to engaging in

behaviors that disrupt sleep. Follow the regime on which you and your sleep specialist collaborate.

SLEEP TO YOUR HEALTH

Sleep and health are interdependent. Volumes of scientific studies in this area have identified the association between poor sleep and illness or medical disorders, including but not limited to cardiovascular disease, gastrointestinal disorder, increased health complaints, and emotional disorders.

The World Health Organization stated that health includes in its definition components of mental, social, and physical factors. To date, there is a paucity of research investigating how people feel about their health or their level of well-being. Further investigation is needed that simultaneously looks at these three components (i.e., mental, social, and physical factors) and their relationship to sleep and how satisfied individuals are with their sleep.

REFERENCES

1. Partinen, M., Patkonen, P.T.S., Kaprio, J., Koskenvuo, N., & Hilakiv, I. (1982). Sleep disorders in relation to coronary heart disease. *Acta Medica Scandinavica, 660* (Suppl.), 123–136.
2. Hyppa, M. T., & Kronholm, F. (1989). Quality of sleep and chronic illness. *Journal of Clinical Epidemiology, 42,* 633–638.
3. Phillips, B., Mayan, L., Gerhardstein, C., & Cecil, B. (1991). Shift work, sleep quantity and worker health: A study of police officers. *Southern Medical Journal, 84,* 1176–1197.
4. Pilcher, J. J., Ginter, D. R., & Sadowski, B. (1996). Sleep quality versus sleep quantity: Relationships between sleep and measures of health, well-being and sleepiness in college students. *Journal of Psychosomatic Research, 42*(6), 583–596.

MENOPAUSE AND POOR SLEEP

Women are more likely to use organizers or calendars to track their schedules. They are also more likely to have written goals. When women have free time, they are more likely to read or do household chores than are males.[1] When unexpected events occur, women are more likely to experience sleep disturbance in the form of insomnia. As a result, excessive daytime sleepiness and fatigue prevail.

Hot flashes (vasomotor flushing) are one of the most common perimenopausal symptoms. These symptoms generally occur between the ages of 45 and 55 years. Vasomotor flushing occurs throughout the day and night without trackable cause and is often the most disturbing symptom experienced by menopausal women. Other physiological symptoms can also occur, such as increased heart rate, tingling in hands, and nausea. The etiology of hot flashes is due to the lower levels of estrogen in the body, and treatment has focused on estrogen replacement therapy. Using estrogen replacement therapy has a major side effect on sleep, however; it can precipitate or aggravate an existing sleep disturbance into a full-blown sleep disorder. Unfortunately, in some cases, women have to choose between the benefits of estrogen replacement and the deleterious effects (i.e., difficulty falling and/or staying asleep, which are insomnia complaints) on sleep. Additionally, changes in diet can affect the number and intensity of hot flashes.[2]

Furthermore, night sweats can also fragment and worsen sleep, not to mention the emotional effect they have on many women. The collection of menopausal symptoms (e.g., hot flashes, nighttime sweating, mood changes, etc.) often promotes change in women's lives. Women may choose to change their actions (e.g., cool their body temperature by stopping what they are doing, changing clothes and/or temperature settings) or how they respond to hot flashes, but night sweats are often problematic and less easy to manage. Nighttime sweating episodes are caused by declining estrogen levels and can be *very* disruptive to sleep. A night of sleep becomes fragmented by night sweats, which arouse the sleeper to wakefulness, sometimes several times throughout the night. The end result, a night of fragmented sleep, leaves the woman waking up unrefreshed and often sleepy throughout the day. Sleepiness can also lead to changes in mood, energy, cognitive functioning, and performance. It is hard to feel like you are on top of your game if you are sleepy.

Night sweats are not the only menopausal symptom plaguing women. Excessive sleepiness and more florid dreaming result from too much progesterone. Self-report data on this topic revealed equivalent frustration when comparing these two types of menopausal symptoms, with night sweating having a lowered overall severity rating.[2]

It is ironic that treatments for menopausal symptoms often seem like some new experimental method for a newly discovered phenomenon rather than an age-old fact of life. Good research in this area is at an early developmental stage compared to intervention studies. Interventions have been identified, but efficiency of these interventions needs to be documented. Specifically, more research needs to explore the following factors: exercise to increase blood circulation, relaxation to decrease nervous system arousal, estrogen replacement therapy to moderate declining estrogen levels, nutritional assessment and diet change to affect metabolic change, and a myriad of alternative care therapies (including herbal medicines) to determine the overall effectiveness on reducing menopausal symptoms. What we do know for certain is that if you improve your sleep, you will feel better. This statement may be difficult for women experiencing significant symptoms, but finding the most effective intervention will reduce symptoms and sleep will improve.

IMPORTANT INFORMATION FOR PERIMENOPAUSAL WOMEN

With the onset of menopause and the changes in hormones (predominantly estrogen), there generally is an increase in weight. The effect of increasing body weight and sleep are quite known. When we gain weight (for both men and women), this change in body composition places us at greater risk of experiencing sleep-related breathing disorders (e.g., sleep apnea), which cause us to have more restless and fragmented nights of sleep. How do we combat the increase in weight commonly experienced by menopausal women? Exercise. Exercise is needed not only to increase blood circulation but also to fight obesity. We also know that exercise, if done four to six hours before bedtime, increases slow-wave sleep. Furthermore, a number of research studies have identified a link between obesity and insulin resistance, leading to type 2 diabetes.[2] Such metabolic disorders may occur for some with the body shape changes that may occur with age-related weight gain (i.e., two pounds a year after age 40), particularly if the weight gain is in the stomach area rather than in the hips.

Unfortunately, many menopausal women may experience cognitive and mood changes. Symptoms can include a waning in attention and concentration. An adequate sleep duration becomes essential for menopausal and perimenopausal women to provide opportunity for REM (dreaming occurs in REM). This REM time builds opportunity for new learning of information. Most important, loss of sleep negatively affects mood, personality, and cognitive functioning. Sleep can reverse these negative effects and improve overall quality of life for menopausal women.

The following are examples of things that we can do to improve mood and sleep:

1. Utilizing bright-light therapy increases the flow of melatonin and is recommended for improving sleep and mood; however, using bright lights should be done only under the instruction of a sleep therapist.
2. Reducing eating large, heavy meals at bedtime or close to bedtime serves the purpose of avoiding gastric reflux, a common malady that can come with advancing age. It is also important to monitor the type of food (e.g., fatty meats and food containing large amounts of sugars and/or carbohydrates) being consumed.

REFERENCES

1. Daytimer. Survey on adults and their time. Retrieved June 6, 2006 from http://www.daytimer.com/timemanagementresources.
2. Northrup, C. (2001). *The wisdom of menopause.* New York: Bantam Books.

EMOTIONS AND POOR SLEEP

It is likely that you have heard about the relationship between chronic poor sleep and one's emotions in the news. We have all experienced one or more night of poor sleep and noticed the negative effect it had on our emotions. There is a plethora of research suggesting that persistent insomnia leads to depression.[1] Some of these studies revealed that the appearance of sleep disturbance may be a preceding factor to depression. Further investigation into this area needs to be conducted, however, because we can only say that there is a relationship or association between insomnia and depression. At this point, scientists cannot say that persistent insomnia causes depression.

Sleep disturbances cause changes in health. Individuals experiencing minor health conditions (e.g., colds, flus, aches, and pains) to major concerns (e.g., uncontrolled diabetes) experience the world differently. The ability to rest, relax, and sleep is altered. This sleep alteration, commonly experienced as fragmented sleep, influences a person's health status. For example, sleep-laboratory studies have measured changes in sleep in patients with depression.[2] Several features of sleep are altered in depressed patients, including total sleep time, time to fall asleep, and distribution of each sleep stage. Young adults with depression diagnoses tend to have increased sleep periods and shortened time to fall asleep. Additionally, research studies have also identified that depressed patients also enter into dream sleep (REM) faster than nondepressed patients. In other words, depressed patients quickly enter into REM and have decreased time spent in NREM (deep sleep is decreased).[3] This lowered amount of deep sleep has been found to be related to reoccurrence of symptoms. The abnormal sleep architecture (i.e., stages and percentages of NREM and REM are altered) in those with depression has also been identified in those at risk for depression. If you feel that you are depressed or have a family history or past history of depression and are experiencing sleep disturbance, please schedule an appointment with a sleep specialist.

There are a number of creative interventions to assist improving sleep in depressed patients. Therapeutic interventions vary from neurotransmitter to pharmacological agents. In historical writings about sleep, purposeful sleep deprivation was prescribed by Hippocrates to serve as a reset for the body when poor sleep and headache pain prevailed. By current standards, this may have worked because it altered the person's sleep architecture and corresponding biochemistry. Again, it is important to consult with a sleep specialist if you are experiencing depression and sleep disturbance.

In extreme emotionally disordered conditions such as Alzheimer's disease, Parkinson's disease, and schizophrenia, the patterning of the sleep-wake cycle and sleep architecture is significantly altered. Sleep periods and types of sleep periods (i.e., REM or NREM) are chaotic. In general, the person's sleep rhythms are disordered secondary to biochemical changes in the disorder affecting the biochemistry of the sleep cycle. The individual with these types of illness loses the ability to regulate the sleep-wake cycle so that sleepiness and alertness occur at inappropriate times.

Sleep specialists have expert training in this area. Their clinical training and background will ensure an accurate diagnosis of emotional disorders and provide workable pathways to address and improve the sleep alterations. Family members are often included in learning about the treatment protocol. They are also educated about the emotional disorder and the appropriate treatment so that there is a greater understanding of the disorder and the necessary changes needed to improve their loved one's sleep.

If a sleep specialist is consulted, the patient may have to spend the night at a sleep laboratory for a nighttime sleep study followed by a daytime nap study. These sleep studies will provide a precise measure of the patient's sleep and provide the necessary information as to what actually occurs during nighttime and daytime sleep. Furthermore, depending on the symptoms, a sleep log may also be requested, which will provide a subjective measure of sleep. The sleep specialist will likely work in consultation with the referring clinician and/or psychiatrist to actively monitor the patient's emotional and sleep changes, especially if pharmaceutical agents have been prescribed. Last, the sleep specialist will request follow-up visits to ensure and encourage that the recommended changes are being implemented.

REFERENCES

1. Breslau, N., Roth, T., Rosenthal, L., & Andreski, P. (1996). Sleep disturbance and psychiatric disorders: A longitudinal epidemiological study of young adults. *Biological Psychiatry, 39*(6), 411–418.
2. Hall, M. D., Buysse, D. J., Reynolds, III, C. F., Kupfer, D. J., & Baum, A. (1996). Stress related intrusive thoughts disrupt sleep onset and contiguity. *Journal of Sleep Research, 25,* 163.
3. Perlis, M. L., Giles, D. E., Buysse, D. J., Tu, X., & Kupfer, D. J. (1997). Self-reported sleep disturbance as a prodromal symptom in recurrent depression. *Journal of Affective Disorder, 42,* 309–312.

DREAMING PROBLEMS AND OTHER SUCH MATTERS

During the seven or so hours, on average, that we typically sleep, we have several dream episodes. Approximately five dream episodes, or rapid eye movement (REM) sleep, occur. The term *REM sleep* is based on the quick left to right movements of the eyeball that occur during REM sleep. We often hear people report that they do not dream; everyone dreams, however, but some individuals just do not recall their dreams. Dream recall usual occurs if there is an awakening for more than a couple of seconds. If this type of awakening occurs, we are more likely to remember a dream or part of a dream.

REM sleep is distinctly different from non-REM (NREM) sleep. Each REM period provides a different set of physiological events compared to NREM sleep. During REM sleep, heart rate, blood flow and pressure are increased, the rhythm of breathing is changed, and body temperature cannot be regulated. This type of acceleration of the nervous system is prompted by biochemical changes in the brain's activity during REM as compared to NREM.

The brain during REM sleep releases neurotransmitters that maintain this sleep stage. Neurotransmitters generate connections to other nearby structures in the brain. Essentially, neurotransmitters communicate to other structures in the brain, and this communication causes various changes. For example, due to this communication, there is a reduction in muscle activity throughout the body (except for the eyes), commonly referred to as muscle paralysis. Reduced muscle activity and muscle paralysis are normal occurrences in REM sleep. A small percentage (less than 10%) of the time, these physiological events occur in NREM sleep.

A complete sleep cycle (experiencing Stages 1 through 4 and REM sleep) occurs every 90 minutes. The brain activity and biochemical changes are synchronized to the sleep-wake schedule in a rhythmic fashion.[1] Awakenings from sleep and from various stages of sleep may occur due to certain medications or recreational substances (i.e., drugs and alcohol) or if an individual is experiencing stress.

The term *nightmare,* or *nachtmar,* comes from a combination of French and Latin (*nacht,* or "night," and *mar,* or "spirit"). It is used to refer to the state of awakening from NREM (slow wave) sleep. Generally, individuals do *not* experience nightmares in REM sleep. When a person experiences REM sleep, by convention, they will experience dreams, dream anxiety attacks, and drug-induced dreams.[2] An abrupt awakening from REM sleep with moderate nervous system activity (i.e., increased heart rate, shortness of breath) is a dream anxiety attack. The dreamer, here, may or may not remember the events, and the content of the dream does include feelings of oppression, domination, or cruelty. Some medication may bring forth more dreaming or more florid dreaming. These classes of medications generally include antidepressants, antihypertensives, and anti-Parkinsonians.[2] Last, dreaming is a natural state, and the first time you dream will occur about one-and-a-half hours after you fall asleep. On average, we experience approximately four episodes of REM per nighttime sleep.

Analyze Your Dreams

1. Traditional approaches look for symbolic meanings for each aspect of the dream. Try to determine how the content of your dream mimics or symbolizes what is happening in your life.

2. Consider yourself a playwright; the dream researcher Calvin Hall encourages analysis of setting, case, and emotions.

3. Think scientifically; the dream researcher Rosalind Cartwright suggested looking logically at the emotional tone of dream followed by a determination of what events or circumstances contributed to this tone. This type of thinking is followed by planning possible alternative behaviors or outcomes during your wake day that you may consider to deter that tone.

4. Lucid dreaming is when the dreamer is awake and able to have normal thought and action. Researchers use this approach in a laboratory setting in which sleep is recorded, as are the person's comments.

5. Most important to remember: You have control of the outcome of your dreams. If you experience an unpleasant or frightening dream and you wake up, go back into the dream even if you cannot return to sleep and create the outcome that you want. These actions will promote feelings of control and empowerment.

Record Your Dreams[1]

1. Be purposeful in recording your dreams by planning which nights and how you will do this. It is most straightforward if you keep a pad of paper and a pen at bedside.

2. When you awaken in the morning, try not to move about too much and write down everything. Do not worry about grammar, spelling, or neatness—just write.

3. Although this may sound funny, try to write down all that comes to mind with your eyes closed.

4. Reread what you wrote, then write down any other details.

5. Keep all the dreams recorded in the same place.

The themes of dreams are as varied as human nature. These techniques of dream analysis may be helpful in analysis of your dreams.

REM SLEEP ABNORMALITIES

For some people, abnormalities in REM sleep may occur. Of more serious concern are the REM disorders, including sleep paralysis, hypnagogic hallucinations, and REM behavior disorder.[2] In sleep paralysis disorder (also known as RBD), the sleeper's body remains motionless while he regains alertness from his night of sleep. This can be dangerous because individuals can act out their dreams and hurt themselves or someone else (most likely their bed partner). Hypnagogic hallucinations are defined as strange and oftentimes scary dreamlike experiences while falling asleep.[2]

REM behavior disorder (RBD) has received a lot of attention in the popular press. During REM sleep, the muscles become paralyzed during sleep and can oscillate between being paralyzed and somewhat paralyzed during sleep. In RBD, however, there is an aberrant change in the active inhibition of motor activity. What does this statement mean? The sleeper loses the ability to remain paralyzed during REM sleep, and during dreams he literally acts out dreams. For example, an elderly patient was a prisoner of war survivor and was having a dream that he was fighting during the Vietnam War. Typically, the dreamer should be paralyzed so that he remains in bed and does not act out the dream. This patient was able to act out his dreams and once dove off of his bed because he was dreaming that he was diving into a river. He ended up having to go to the emergency room because of multiple face fractures and bodily injuries. Although RBD is not common, when detected it can be successfully treated with medication and scheduling of the sleep period.

REFERENCES

1. Cartwright, R. (1977). *Night life exploration in dreaming.* Englewood Cliffs, NJ: Prentice Hall.
2. Mahowald, M. W., & Schenck, C. H. (2000). Diagnosis and management of parasomnias. *Clinical Cornerstone, 2*(5), 48–57.

YOUR HEALTH AND YOUR SLEEP

The importance of good sleep contributing to good health has been known for centuries. The National Sleep Alert[1] placed the focus on improving sleep quality with documented evidence of its impact on cardiovascular, musculoskeletal, pulmonary, endocrine, and immunological functioning. At minimum, in effect, poor sleep worsens already poor health, and in general it negatively influences risk factors for disease and other types of medical disorders.

The shifting of biochemical actions in the brain during various stages of sleep and the alternating patterns of brain wave activity, as with any biological system, are interrelated to other systems. The four major categories of sleep disturbance—insomnias, hypersomnias, parasomnias, and sleep-wake schedule disorders—are often undiagnosed. This lack of attention to sleep disorders is particularly relevant when an individual already has a medical condition. The complication of sleep disturbance worsens the symptomology for that individual. For instance, an 81-year-old patient was referred for excessive daytime sleepiness by his family practitioner. This referral came from a practitioner he just switched to because his former internist (whom he had seen for more than 25 years) had never suggested that he see a sleep specialist. This patient had a significant medical history; most pertinent was his cardiac history. He experienced four heart attacks, with his second heart attack rendering him disabled at the age of 58 years old. His wife accompanied him to the appointment, and she stated that he snored loudly, even when sitting in a chair, and she was often scared because he looked like he stopped breathing during the night. She stated that he slept this way for approximately thirty years. A nighttime sleep study revealed that he had severe obstructive sleep apnea. He was appropriately treated with a CPAP (continuous positive airway pressure) mask and reported feeling more alert and having more energy than he had in years. He actually stated, "I feel alive again." It is unfortunate that clinicians often let sleep disorders go undiagnosed or neglect asking questions about sleep.

In fact, the Sleep Heart Health Study completed in 2001 identified the association between sleep-disordered breathing and self-reported cardiovascular disease. Results from this large-scale study indicated a relationship between hypertension, coronary artery disease, and congestive heart failure with sleep-disordered breathing. Once detected in a sleep study, patients with sleep-disordered breathing are treated with CPAP, in which air is released into the throat while wearing a mask to enhance this effect. Reductions in blood pressure have been observed for a very brief period following the CPAP treatment (i.e., within five days).[2] When a patient is able to reduce his weight, rates of sleep-disordered breathing are substantially reduced. Weight reduction can be a key variable in reducing risks of sleep-related breathing disorders.

Sleep specialists commonly inquire about daytime sleepiness. It is essential to distinguish sleepiness from fatigue. Sleepiness relates to the ability or propensity to fall asleep. Fatigue refers to physical weakness and tiredness, usually related to exertion. If, however, the fatigue is not corresponding to activity, the source of lethargy is often related to emotional mood. Depression is associated with sleep disturbance. Overnight sleep studies followed by a daytime nap studies assist in identifying between sleepiness and fatigue. With sleep-disordered breathing and subsequent daytime sleepiness, nighttime breathing patterns are carefully monitored during nighttime sleep studies. In fact, pulmonary disease is prevalent, and reports of more than 60 percent of these individuals awaken throughout the night due to asthma attacks.[3] It may be the case that sleep has a role in nocturnal worsening of poor health, disease, and disorder conditions.

The National Sleep Foundation (NSF) census also reported on the high prevalence of gastric esophageal reflux symptoms at night. Establishing control over these symptoms and preventing frequent awakenings are the keys to successful treatment.[3]

Finally, renal disease is reported by the World Health Organization to be in the top five common chronic illnesses. This high prevalence is accentuated by its correspondence to insomnia and fragmentary sleep. There is also interrelatedness between renal disease, sleep-disordered breathing, restless legs syndrome, and periodic limb movement disorder.

Extreme emotional disorder (i.e., depression, anxiety) has been found to be linked to sleep disturbances of insomnia, excessive sleepiness, abrupt awakenings, and abnormal movements during sleep. In neurological conditions such as Alzheimer's disease, the rhythm of the sleep-wake cycle is altered. A discontinuity of sleep results from this disease.

In some psychiatric conditions, such as schizophrenia, reductions in total sleep time, reductions in amount of REM, and reduced deep sleep occur. Medication prescribed will affect the disordered sleep architecture as well. With regard to depression, if it is seasonally initiated (seasonal affective disorder). The use of bright-light therapy (blue spectrum, >2000 lex) is effective with this condition.[4]

In summary, the most important take-home message is that it is essential to see a sleep specialist to determine if a sleep study is needed in patients with medical conditions and complaints of disordered sleep. Life is far too short and precious to experience disrupted sleep.

REFERENCES

1. National Commission on Sleep Disorder Research. (1993). *Wake up America: A national sleep alert: Vol. 1. Executive summary and executive report.* Bethesda, MD: National Institutes of Health.
2. Becker, H. F., Jerrentrup, A., Ploch, T., Grote, L., Penzel, T., Sullivan, C. E., et al. (2003). Effect of nasal continuous positive airway pressure treatment on blood pressure in patients with obstructive sleep apnea. *American Journal of Respiratory Critical Care Medicine, 107,* 68–73.
3. National Sleep Foundation. (2006). *National Sleep Foundation sleep survey.* Washington, DC: National Sleep Foundation.
4. Terman, M., Terman, J. S., Ee-sing, L., & Cooper, T. B. (2001). Circadian time of morning light administration and therapeutic response in winter depression. *Archives of General Psychiatry, 58,* 69–75.

FURTHER READING

Ancoli-Israel, S., Kripke, D. F., Klauber, H. R., Mason W. J., Fell, R., & Kaplan, O. (1991). Sleep-disordered breathing in community dwelling elderly. *Sleep, 14,* 486–495.

Edgar, D. (1996). Circadian control of sleep/wakefulness: Implications in shift work and therapeutic. In K. Shirak, S. Sagawa, & M. Yousef (Eds.), *Physiological basis of occupational health: Stressful environments* (pp. 253–265). Amsterdam: SPB Academic Publishing.

Kapur, U. K., Redline, S., Nieto, F. J., Young, T. B., Newman, A. B., & Henderson, J. A.. (2002). The relationship between chronically disrupted sleep and health care use. *Sleep, 25*(3), 289–296.

SLEEPY ATHLETES

It has been suggested that deep sleep serves as a time for the body to physically restore itself. The activities of the immune and endocrine systems are at their best functioning during deep sleep. For instance, new cells to combat disease are generated during deep sleep.

Exercise has been associated with affecting deep sleep. Some reports have indicated that exercise increases deep sleep. It is not the case that exercise enhances deep sleep in so much that it enhances sleep in general. Regular exercise increases circulation and promotes respiratory efficiency, which in turn promotes a regular sleep pattern.

The athlete's experience of exercise and sleep is much more intense. The effort put forth during workouts and competitions also affect the quality and quantity of sleep. Although exercise can have beneficial effects of deepening sleep, athletes can also experience sleep disturbance.

Sleep loss is the most common sleep disturbance experienced by athletes. The apprehension before an event may cause sleeplessness in an athlete. The outcome of this apprehension is that sleep tends to be poor, fragmented, and short, which may compromise athletic performance, not to mention the possibility of incurring an injury.

The timing of workouts can sometimes be problematic on sleep. Early-morning workouts coupled with late-afternoon workouts leaves the athlete fatigued and sleepy. A brief nap of 30 minutes or less may be helpful in recovering from sleepiness, but napping can have a negative influence on sleep. The major effect napping may have on sleep depends on the time the nap is taken. For instance, napping in the early evening may rejuvenate the mind and body enough that when the athlete wants to go to bed, she may not be sleepy.

Furthermore, early-morning sleep disruptions can occur if there is an early departure time for an event. Some athletes report that the traveling itself, with time zone changes and possible climate changes, and the overall strain of adhering to a competition or training schedule are sufficient to disrupt sleep. A brief nap on travel day, especially if the nap occurs in the middle of the day (prior to 3:00 P.M.), may be beneficial in alleviating sleepiness. If the sleep disturbance is more severe, departing earlier and allowing a few days to adjust to a new environment may also be extremely helpful.

In addition to early-morning workouts, sleep may also become disturbed due to muscle soreness. Because of discomfort or pain, sleep may become lightened and fragmented. For example, if you have injured a part of your body, have muscle stiffness, or are in physical pain, lying in bed itself may be painful. Body movements, such as turning during sleep, can awaken the sleeper because of pain or muscle soreness.

Sleep loss affects the amount of Stage 4 sleep. During deep sleep (Stage 4), the endocrine system releases growth hormone, which stimulates muscle growth and repair. Decreased performance occurs in athletes with prolonged sleep loss. Athletes do not and cannot work out as much and cannot sustain a particular intensity of exercise when sleep deprived. For instance, after approximately

36 hours of sleep loss, 10 percent to 11 percent of athletes can experience exhaustion at a moderately hard intensity of about 80%/O_2 max.[1] Sleep loss also reduces coordination and efficiency during exercise.

Body temperature fluctuates within +/– two degrees all day long. Exercise increases body temperature, which in turn promotes the body to cool itself, so there is a compensating drop in body temperature. Thus, exercise, in effect, regulates sleep because we need our body temperatures low at the start of sleep. Too much exercise, however, as in the case of athletes with double workouts, can cause sleep loss because the body is too hot to be able to fall asleep. Body temperature also rises more quickly when the athlete is sleep deprived. In sum, if your body temperature is too hot or cold, sleep initiation will be difficult. Have you ever tried falling asleep on a very hot evening during summer? If you have, you most likely recall the difficulty you experienced.

GENERAL SLEEP GUIDELINES FOR ATHLETES

1. During away competitions, place together athletes with similar sleep schedules as roommates.
2. Where possible, give athletes a choice for the second part of their workout (i.e., lifting on their own time).
3. Varying the practice time and tracking feedback from athletes will assist in identifying when the athletes are at their optimal time to perform physically, mentally, and socially.

REFERENCE

1. Luenstein, R., & Galehouse, D. (2004). *The making of a student athlete*. Peak Performance Newsletter. Retrieved October 19, 2006, from https://www.pperformance.com

WORK AND SLEEP

It is the work of Thomas Edison and his invention of the light-bulb that has frequently been identified as causing individuals to stay awake longer, because the lightbulb extended the workday. Approximately 400 workers were surveyed about their sleep, work schedule, and health, and undiagnosed (but self-perceived) sleep problems were commonly reported.[1] Furthermore, a comparison of all the questions responded to on the survey indicated an association between perceived sleep problems and general health maladies. Interestingly, survey questions regarding work, such as satisfaction, performance, and absenteeism, were related to reported sleep problems.[1]

Within the last thirty years, approximately 158 hours annually (about a month of work) has been added to the work schedule.[2] This estimate includes commute time, and this addition of work hours during the day actually subtracts hours from sleep time.

In general, workers with poor sleep also report health, general functioning, and well-being as being compromised. Additionally, workers reporting sleep disturbance also describe experiencing a reduction in energy and vitality. It is unfortunate that workers, as a group, tend to report sleep disturbance and corresponding disturbance in daytime functioning, yet they often do not seek help for their sleep problems. Workers will often push through the day, have excessive absences, and use over-the-counter medicines.[1]

Because a large proportion of the working population reports experiencing sleep disturbance (per self-report), workers are encouraged to schedule an appointment with a sleep specialist. A sleep specialist will conduct an assessment, and perhaps the worker will be required to complete some questionnaires that will provide a more in-depth look at the disturbance.

It is necessary to identify sleepiness in workers, and it becomes even more important for those with jobs necessitating constant vigilance and/or working in hazardous environments. The magnitude of danger secondary to human error caused by sleepiness is substantial. For example, the *Exxon Valdez* accident was due to one barge crashing into another, causing a significant oil spill that was hazardous to wildlife and endangered many species of animals. Other accidents of enormous magnitude (e.g., the Three Mile Island power plant) have been identified with sleepiness related to ongoing sleep deprivation. Military workers and medical and safety professionals are but a few members of the workforce for whom sleepiness resulting from an undiagnosed sleep disturbance has the propensity to have deleterious affects on a significant number of people.[3] Because we do not know the exact nature of sleep disturbance in the working population, estimates have suggested that approximately 29 percent experience sleep disorders. Estimates are that 70 million Americans have excessive daytime sleepiness.[4]

The extent of compromised work functioning secondary to sleep disturbance has been related to excessive sleepiness, work-related accidents, low work performance and satisfaction, absenteeism, and performance degradation. The table on the following page provides some strategies in assisting the worker in gaining relief from disturbed sleep.

Human Body Temperature and Sleep Cycle

Worker Problem	Strategy
Excessive daytime sleepiness	Scheduled brief daytime naps (30 minutes or less and before 3 pm)
Work performance decrements	Obtain core amount of sleep per night (at least 7 hours) with regular bedtimes and wake times
Difficulty with attention and concentration	Consistent sleep period each day; abstain from excessive caffeine—mild to moderate use only
Mood changes and/or accidents at work related to sleepiness	See sleep specialist to collaboratively develop problem solving plan. Stress management is needed
Fatigue (tiredness, not sleepiness)	Relaxation, calm setting for at least 30 minutes to physically rest—maintain sitting position

During the on-the-job time when sleepiness may be problematic, use strategies to create elevated attention and perseverance. Although not solutions to a sleep disturbance problem, small measures such as actively engaging in conversation or walking up stairs or taking a brief break and walking for 5 to 10 minutes can stimulate thinking. This action will give the brain a message to be involved in thinking and problem solving rather than relaxation and eventual sleep.

Second, as previously explained in chapter 2, when we fall asleep, our natural circadian rhythm keeps us asleep. Approximately three hours after we fall asleep, melatonin is released, which enhances sleep physiologically (it helps us to stay asleep longer). Light is the most powerful and natural regulator of sleep, and there is a direct relationship between light exposure and melatonin release.[5] Obtaining as much natural bright light in the early-morning hours and/or in early afternoon will accentuate this cycle. *Do not obtain bright-light exposure within several hours of bedtime or during the night. Exposure during these inappropriate times will promote alertness.* These strategies and tactics are just a temporary measure for the worker to utilize until a thorough assessment is conducted by a sleep specialist. Last, for those workers trying to recover from jet lag, the use of early-morning light may be helpful, but we strongly urge them to consult with a sleep specialist.

REFERENCES

1. Kupperman, M., Lubek, D. P., Mazonson, P. D., Patrick, D. L., Steward, A. L., Buesching, D. P., et al. (1995). Sleep problems and their correlates in a working population. *Journal of General Internal Medicine, 10,* 25–32.
2. Dement, W. C., & Vaughan, C. (2000). *The promise of sleep: A pioneer in sleep medicine explores the vital connection between health, happiness, and a good night's sleep.* New York: Dell Publishing.
3. Johnson, L. C., & Spinweber, C. L. (1983). Good and poor sleepers differ in Navy performance. *Military Medicine, 148,* 727–731.
4. National Commission on Sleep Disorder Research. (1993). *Wake up America: A national sleep alert: Vol. 1. Executive summary and executive report.* Bethesda, MD: National Institutes of Health.
5. Ehret, C. F., & Scanlon, L. W. (1983). *Overcoming jet lag.* New York: Berkley.

FURTHER READING

Baeher, E. K., Fogg, L. F., & Eastman, C. I. (1999). Intermittent bright light and exercise to entrain human circadian rhythms to night work. *American Journal of Physiology, 177*(6, Pt. 2), R1598–1604.
Beers, T. (2000). Flexible schedules and shift work: Replacing the 9 to 5 workday? *Monthly Labor Review, 123,* 33–40.
Knutsson, A. (2003). Health disorders of shift workers. *Occupational Medicine, 53,* 103–108.

Leger, D. (1993). The prevalence of jet-lag among 507 traveling business-men. *Sleep Research, 22,* 409.

Presser, H. (2003). *Working is a 24/7 economy: Challenges for American families.* New York: Russell Sage Foundation.

Purnell, M. T., Feyer, A. M., & Herbison, G. P. (2002). The impact of a nap opportunity during the night shift on the performance and alertness of 12h shift worker. *Journal of Sleep Research, 11*(3), 219–227.

Summala, H., & Mikkola, T. (1994). Fatal accidents among car and truck drivers: Effects of fatigue, age and alcohol consumption. *Human Factors, 36,* 315.

Walsh, J. K., Muehlbac, M. J., & Schweitzer, P. K., (1995). Hypnotics and caffeine as countermeasure for shift work-related sleepiness and sleep disturbance. *Journal of Sleep Research, 4*(S2), 80–83.

HEALTHY PRACTICES AND
YOUR SLEEP

Alternative medicine practices have surged in popularity. They have tremendous accessibility to the consumer and varying degrees of satisfaction. Although little research substantiates the positive claims of effectiveness, their use continues. These practices referred to are called, collectively, *complementary* and *alternative medicine.*

Mind-body therapies such as acupuncture, massage therapy, and music therapy provide soothing guides to relaxation. This state allows for deep breathing, enhanced blood circulation, and relaxed muscle tone. The result is often immediate. There is some research in this area to suggest that the expectation that something will work may actually work, due not to the efficacy of the therapy but rather due to the so-called placebo effect. A placebo is an inert substance that cannot produce any change in an experiment because it is powerless, but the person or participant believes it to be powerful and therefore will report changes as if the placebo really was an agent capable of producing change.

The natural remedies of herbal medicine and aromatherapy have widespread appeal. Physician monitoring is essential here. Several herbs, including chamomile tea and lavender essential oil, are examples of natural remedies used to help insomnia. Sleep hygiene practices include the use of a constant sleep pattern (i.e., regular wake-up time and bedtime) and limited caffeine use. In general, sleep hygiene practices have considerable heterogeneity with respect to the sleeper. That is to say, a wide variety of sleepers utilize this type of sleep hygiene factor with moderate success. In effect, maintaining a regular bedtime and wake-up time provides a stable, consistent message to the brain as to the need for activity.

This pacemaker role of sleep uncovered by fundamental studies in this area underscores the importance of maintaining regular sleep periods.[1,2] These cycles of activity of hormone release, growth hormone being one of them, are interdependent to the sleep-wake cycle.[2] Thus, your regular bedtime and wake time behaviorally punctuate a predictable schedule upon which other systems of the body depend.

Caffeine is a common drink that many individuals drink throughout the day; however it is an altering (e.g., stimulating) substance that can disturb sleep. Although caffeine can be alerting or stimulating when consumed strategically, it is disruptive to sleep when used throughout the day. Specifically, caffeine consumption should begin approximately one hour before times of expected decreased daytime alertness. Caffeine consumption should stop about three hours before bedtime and much longer than that in individuals sensitive to the alerting and addictive effects (e.g., the elderly). Also, caffeine is a diuretic and can lead to dehydration, particularly if individuals are in a low-humidity setting (e.g., work in an enclosed office).

Caffeine is found in many substances, such as tea, coffee, cola, and a number of medicines (e.g., Excedrin). It is commonly ingested upon awakening, due to its alerting effects. Caffeine has an alerting effect on sleep inertia. Sleep inertia is reduced cognitive performance, grogginess, and tendency to return to sleep. In addition to the subjective or individual dissatisfaction with feeling the sleepiness of sleep inertia, it may also place a person in danger if her work or activities require a high level of performance. Caffeine works in promoting alertness because it activates the chemistry in the brain to block one of the chemicals thought to be involved in sleep (adenosine).[1] With sleep inertia intensifying with sleep loss, we can see why caffeine consumption is so popular (e.g., long lines at the zillions of Starbucks and Caribou Coffee shops around the country).

REFERENCES

1. Dement, W. C., & Vaughan, C. (2000). *The promise of sleep: A pioneer in sleep medicine explores the vital connection between health, happiness, and a good night's sleep.* New York: Dell Publishing.
2. Wegscheider, H. J. (1992). *The light book.* Los Angeles: Jeremy P. Tarcher.

SHOULD YOU TRY MELATONIN PILLS FROM THE HEALTH FOOD STORE?

Although sales of melatonin pills exceed sales of vitamins, the health and sleep benefits from melatonin are unfounded. Melatonin's main function is to coordinate circadian rhythms. An experienced sleep specialist may use melatonin with jet-lag patients while carefully monitoring their sleep. Melatonin has also been used in the treatment of seasonal affective disorder and in shift workers. In both situations, the scientific reasoning justifying melatonin to alleviate symptoms is unfounded. In summary, further investigation into the use of melatonin to treat sleep disturbance, specifically at what appropriate dosage and its potential side effects (e.g., cardiac) on human beings, is necessary. We strongly advise against anyone not under the direction of a sleep specialist to take melatonin to assist with sleep.

Source: Bonn, D. (1996). Melatonin's multifarious marvels: Miracle or myth? *The Lancet, 347,* 184.

SHOULD YOUR PET SLEEP WITH YOU?

There is little research on this broadly popular topic of pets sleeping with their owners. One estimate in this area indicated that 80 percent of patients (who were pet owners) in a sleep lab had their pets sleep with them.

When pets sleep on the bed with their owner(s), they disrupt sleep. Potential awakenings due to the pet's movements, noises (e.g., barking), snoring, need to go outside, and increased temperature from body heat may awaken the owner and thereby fragment their sleep. Despite the potential for pets to disrupt their owner's sleep, many pet owners sacrifice the quality and quantity of the sleep in exchange for being close to their pet.

This situation may be complicated by pet owners with allergies. For instance, the owner may be allergic to the pet's dander, and the pet sleeping on or in the bed, especially on the pillows, can aggravate allergies. Also, pet owners on CPAP machines or other health care machines are at risk for some interference of the instruments' functions with a cat or dog climbing around the wiring or machine to get into bed.

Source: Shephard, J. Medical director of Mayo Clinic Sleep Disorders Center.

FOOD AND SLEEP

There are no magic foods to promote sleep. Certain foods at certain times may cause mild sleepiness for some individuals, but food on its own as a single variable to produce sleep is not enough. What does work on sleep and has been scientifically proved is healthy eating.

Nutritional assessments involve a thorough analysis of your weight, eating habits, types of foods consumed, and the timing (when you eat) of foods. This type of food intake analysis can be conducted by a licensed dietician or nutritionist and will assist in learning about how to maintain a balanced diet.

In a Nutrition 101 class, you learn that all energy is provided by three classes of nutrients: fats, carbohydrates, and protein. Other kinds of nutrients are consumed as well: vitamins and minerals. The Food and Nutrition Board of the National Academy of Sciences has determined dietary reference intakes, which are the amounts of nutrients needed for optimal health and to prevent deficiencies. For proper energy and good health, the amount of food (calories) consumed needs to equal energy expended.

When we eat, the digestion process of four hours or more involves the production of heat, as much as 30 percent higher than our resting metabolic level. Over the course of the day, it is estimated that heat generated by food digestion is about 5 percent to 10 percent of total energy expenditure.

You may see in the popular literature suggestions of foods to increase the natural production of the brain chemical serotonin, which is associated with sleep. In general, these diets recommend the intake of carbohydrates (complex, such as rice, potatoes, pasta) that are chemically converted through a series of chemical reactions in the body to generate serotonin.[1] Synthetic or manufactured substances, such as L-tryptophan, mimic this series of chemical reactions that produce serotonin in the brain. L-tryptophan has been found to be dangerous and is not supported, although its popularity carries on. We *do not* recommend that anyone ingest L-tryptophan.

Melatonin manufactured into tablets can be purchased at any local drug store and has also been investigated as a so-called sleep pill. Foods such as oats, sweet corn, rice, Japanese radishes, ginger, tomatoes, bananas, and barley contain melatonin.[2] We have already discussed melatonin and its effect on sleep; we wanted you to be aware that melatonin can also be found in foods (see table below).

What is one to conclude with the myriad messages about foods and sleep? Maintain a balanced diet. Yes, maintain a balanced diet of foods to give you optimal health. Too much of one food group,

Foods Containing Serotonin

Avocado	Eggplant	Pineapple
Banana	Papaya	Plantain banana
Dates	Passion fruit	Walnuts

Source: Pennington, J.A.T. (1989). *Bowe's and Church's: Food values of portions commonly used.* Philadelphia: J. B. Lippincott.

say of protein, may be upsetting to your stomach and give you symptoms of gastrointestinal upset. Gastrointestinal upset disrupts sleep with frequent awakenings because digestion during sleep may involve having the food reverse itself back up the esophagus. It is best to stay away from quick fixes or snacks containing large amounts of carbohydrates and refined sugars generally found in candy bars, pastries, and so forth. Although they may produce a transient increase in alertness (the so-called sugar high) as they are digested, a decrease in alertness or sleepiness may occur.[3] Last, eating a diet high in carbohydrates and fats promote weight gain. Weight gain has been associated with sleep-related breathing disorders (e.g., obstructive sleep apnea or snoring syndromes). Avoid eating heavy meals prior to bedtime; the digestive process is an energy-producing mechanism, and you may have difficulty trying to fall asleep or remain asleep.

The study of vitamins is rather complex. Fortunately for us, the marketplace has simplified this issue with the generation of multivitamins. The multivitamin meets the necessary requirements by the U.S. Food and Drug Administration and is widely used and economical to obtain. Why use vitamins? Vitamins are large chemical units that are necessary in assisting with chemical reactions in the body.

What do you really need to know about eating a balanced diet and taking vitamins? If you take care of your body and do your best to keep your body healthy by eating well-balanced meals and utilizing multivitamins, your sleep should be positively influenced by your healthy lifestyle, providing you maintain good sleep hygiene and so forth. Furthermore, when alertness is necessary, such as getting up in the early morning to start your day, protein intake will be helpful. When sleepiness is intruding in the middle of the afternoon, simple carbohydrates (such as yogurt, half of a bagel) may be helpful for a short burst of alertness.

REFERENCES

1. Pennington, J.A.T. (1989). *Bowe's and Church's: Food values of portions commonly used.* Philadelphia: J. B. Lippincott.
2. Reiter, R. J., & Robinson, J. (1995). *Melatonin: Your body's natural wonder drug.* New York: Bantam Books.
3. Dinges, D. F., & Broughton, R. J. (Eds.). (1989). *Sleep and alertness: Chronobiological, behavioral, and medical aspects of napping.* New York: Raven.

FURTHER READING

Buxton, O. M., Frank, S. A., L'Hermite-Baleriaux, M., Leproult, R., Turek, F. W. & Van Cauter, E. (1997). Roles of intensity and duration of nocturnal exercise in causing phase delay of human circadian rhythms. *American Journal of Physiology, 273*(3, Pt.1), E536–E542.

Martin, S. K., & Fastman, C. I. (2002). Sleep log of young adults with self-selected sleep times predict the dim light melatonin onset. *Chronobiology International, 19, 695-707.*

National Commission on Sleep Disorder Research. (1993). *Wake up America: A national sleep alert: Vol. 1. Executive summary and executive report.* Bethesda, MD: National Institutes of Health.

CULTURAL INFLUENCES ON SLEEP

Throughout the course of our lives, we gather personal knowledge and competencies to accomplish tasks of life. The manner by which we initiate and proceed in these tasks reflects our social influences, more specifically our culture. These collective so-called ways of knowing are sometimes clearly designated by our race and/or ethnic background, age, and gender. Our thinking is influenced by these social influences and, accordingly, so are our behaviors.

Cultural influences are commonly addressed in the sleep literature in terms of the individual's means of expression. This means of expression means "what we choose to discuss or not to discuss."

One area of sleep in which cultural influences are evident is that of dream content. Based on long-term, careful studies of children, teens, young adults, and adults, age-related differences have been determined. Dream recall ability is low in young children, and it is not until preteen years that their dreams are considered similar to adults in terms of amount recalled, number of characters, and emotions involved.[1] The themes and characters in our dreams also change as we mature in age.

Dream content is often included in religious and medical ceremonies. In this manner, it serves as an inspiration to an action; however, it may vary from culture to culture. The gender difference in dream content with regard to different cultures is similar; across cultures, males have more aggressive dreams involving other males, and females have less aggressive and sexual dreams but more themes involving victimization. Additionally, the mystical incubus, a fiendlike creature that disturbs sleep and aggresses on the defenseless sleeper, is a creation of folklore that is thought to extend from common dream contents of both genders.

Accounts of ethnographic findings across cultures have identified differences in sleep environment, sleep settings, and sleep episodes. In some non-Western cultures, sleeping outdoors, on a platform elevation, or in cave dwellings may be common.[2] Probably the most publicized is the sleep episode that some cultures (e.g., South America, southern Europe) include as a necessary component of daytime: an afternoon nap period, or siesta.[3] The sleep episodes are different by design because some cultures have communal sleeping. The light sleep of the elder is adjacent to the periodic sleep of the infant, which is adjacent to the deep sleep of the school-age child.[2,3] The natural disruption with so many sleep patterns leads to lighter, more fragmented sleep, overall, in these populations.[2,3]

Western society provides a direct contrast to other cultures due to strict beliefs about napping during the day (e.g., it is a sign of laziness and is not productive for employers) and routinization of sleep.[2] Interestingly, in some cultures, sleep has an emotion-regulation function. A type of so-called fear sleep has been described among the Balinese. Documentation of witnesses as well as photos gathered by ethnographers depicts a Balinese thief who fell asleep in the middle of his trial![2] This so-called checking-out function of sleep or a form of escapism is thought to serve an emotional-regulation function.

From a direct, biological basis, there is a racial differential of expression of gene polymorphisms or mutations.[1] Human leukocyte antigens (HLA) are observed in narcolepsy. This gene polymorphism or mutation means that some structural changes occur at the chromosome level to alter the expression of genes. Furthermore, it is believed that there seems to be a so-called timer on the expression of this gene destruction, which unfortunately begins during adolescence (when narcolepsy is commonly diagnosed). However, the level at which the gene destruction occurs and the extent vary between groups of whites, Asians and African Americans.[1] In order to be given a diagnosis of narcolepsy, distinct laboratory tests, including an overnight sleep study, need to be conducted in addition to the information gathered from an interview with a sleep specialist.

REFERENCES

1. Kryger, M. (2005). *Principles and practices of sleep medicine.* New York: Elsevier Press.
2. Worthman, C. M., & Melby, M. K. (2002). Toward a comparative developmental ecology of human sleep. In M. A. Carskadon (Ed.), *Adolescent sleep patterns: Biological, social and psychological influences* (pp. 69–117). New York: Cambridge Press.
3. Androde, M., & Menna-Barreto, L. (2002). Sleep patterns of high school students living in São Paulo, Brazil. In M. A. Carskadon (Ed.), *Adolescent sleep patterns: Biological, social and psychological influences* (pp. 118–131). New York: Cambridge Press.

Appendix

LIFE SPAN ISSUES AND SLEEP

Here is a summary of some possible factors, by age group, that contribute to poor sleep. This matrix is designed from basic scientific literature in the field of sleep medicine. If a section of the matrix seems relevant for you or your family member, then it can become an issue area that you can bring to the attention of your sleep specialist.

Human Sleep Across the Life Span

Age Group	Biological	Emotional	Behavioral/Social	Environmental
Birth-3 months	Periodic sleep	Uses crying if needs are unmet	Comfort with being held, temperature controlled	Noises Temperature comfort
3-6 months	REM/nREM distinct			
6 months-1 year	Differentiation of stages of REM Concentration Arousals		Daytime sleepiness if nap is missed Mood dysregulation	Sleep settings with sleeping alone or with parent
1-5 years			Daytime sleepiness if nap is missed Behavioral excesses if over tired	
6-12 years	Possible nightmare natural if under tension		Behavioral excesses/ over-reacting if sleep deprived Academic problems if sleep deprived and attention concentration an issue	
Teens/Young adulthood	Delayed onset in sleep	Anxiety and tension	Transition to world of work Academic stress from college Relationship	Residential/Coop

Human Sleep Across the Life Span (continued)

Age Group	Biological	Emotional	Behavioral/Social	Environmental
Adulthood 25-50	Insomnia may be problematic if under stress			
Adulthood 50-65	Male often diagnosed at this stage with sleep apnea	Anxiety	Work functioning General health	Schedule constraints
Older adulthood 65+	Advanced sleep schedule Age-related sleep changes of small reduction in sleep length, frequent awakenings to reduced amount of deep sleep Increase in medical conditions: arthritis, pulmonary, gastric reflux that disturb sleep Improper/ excessive use of medications that disturb sleep Over-the-counter medications used	Sadness Bereavement	Retirement Lifestyle changes Napping	Change in home, possibly to residential care Bedroom environment

SLEEP DIARY EXAMPLE

Name:_____ Date:_____

Please place an *X* through every hour (square) that you were able to sleep. If you slept only a half hour during that period, please fill the square with a single diagonal line.

What time did you get up out of bed in the morning?_____
What time did you get into bed in the evening?   _____
Was there anything in particular that woke you this morning (e.g., alarm clock, outside noise, light in window)?   _____

During the day, did you exercise vigorously?
_____ Yes _____ No

If yes, what time of day did you exercise?
_____ Morning   _____ Afternoon   _____ Evening
How long was your exercise session?   _____ minutes
What kind of exercise do you do? _____
_____

Did you drink any beverages or eat any foods that contained caffeine during the 24-hour period (these would include coffee, hot or iced tea, soda pop, chocolate)?
_____ Yes _____ No

If yes, what time of day did you consume these?

a.m.

12-1	1-2	2-3	3-4	4-5	5-6	6-7	7-8	8-9	9-10	10-11	11-12

p.m.

12-1	1-2	2-3	3-4	4-5	5-6	6-7	7-8	8-9	9-10	10-11	11-12

_____ Morning   _____ Afternoon   _____ Evening

How many 8-ounce cups or glasses of caffeinated drinks did you consume? _____

What kind and how much of caffeinated food products did you consume? _____

Did you use nicotine-containing products (cigarettes, snuff, cigars, patch, inhaler, gum) during this period?

_____ Yes _____ No

If yes, what time of day did you use them?

_____ Morning   _____ Afternoon   _____ Evening

How much nicotine did you use (e.g., number of cigarettes or cigars, dosage of patch, etc.)? _____

Did you drink alcohol during this period?

_____Yes _____ No

If yes, what time of day did you drink?

_____ Morning _____ Afternoon _____ Evening

What kind of alcohol do you drink (check all that apply)?

_____ Beer _____ Wine _____ Mixed drinks _____ Liquor

How much did you drink (e.g., number of beers, number of 6-ounce glasses of wine, number of 2-ounce drinks containing liquor)?

Please list all of the medicines (prescribed and over the counter) and other drugs (e.g., cocaine, marijuana) you took in this period.

Medicine or drug	Amount taken	Time of day

MEDIA RESOURCES

CDs

Learn to sleep well: Visualization, music and ocean sounds—The complete aid to a good night's sleep. Duncan Baird.

Mantell, Susie. *Your present: A half-hour of peace.* http://www.relaxintuit.com.

Thompson, Jeffrey. *Delta sleep system: Fall asleep, stay asleep, wake up rejuvenated.* http://www.therelaxationcompany.com.

BOOKS

Carskadon, M. A. (2002). *Adolescent sleep patterns: Biological, social, and psychological influences.* New York: Cambridge Press.

Cartwright, R. D. (1977). *Night life explorations in dreaming.* Englewood Cliffs, NJ: Prentice-Hall.

Cartwright, R., & Lamberg, L. (1992). *Crisis dreaming using your dreams to solve your problems.* New York: HarperCollins Books.

Coren, S. (1996). *Sleep thieves: An eye opening exploration into the science and mysteries of sleep.* New York: Free Press.

Hartman, E. (1987). *The sleep book: Understanding and preventing sleep problems in people over 50.* New York: HarperCollins.

Harvey, J. R. (1998). *Total relaxation: Healing practices for body, mind and spirit.* New York: Kodansha International.

Hauri, P., & Linde, S. (1990). *No more sleepless nights.* New York: Wiley.

Idzikowski, C. (2000). *Learn to sleep well: A practical guide to getting a good night's sleep.* San Francisco: Chronicle Books.

Jouvet, M. (1999). *The paradox of sleep: The story of dreaming.* Boston: MIT Press.

Kryger, M. H. (2004). *A women's guide to sleep disorders.* New York: McGraw-Hill.

Lichstein, K. L., Durrence, H. H., Riedel, B. W., Taylor, D. J., & Bush, A. J. (2004). *Epidemiology of sleep: Age, gender and ethnicity.* Mahwah, NJ: Erlbaum.

Mindell, J. A. (2005). *Sleeping through the night: How infants, toddlers, and their parents can get a good night's sleep.* New York: HarperCollins

Orem, D. A., Reigh, W., Rosenthal, N. E., & Wehr, T. A. (1993). *How to beat jet lag: A practical guide for air travelers.* New York: Henry Holt.

Rosenthal, N. E. (1998). *Winter blues seasonal affective disorder: What it is and how to overcome it.* New York: Guilford.

Sexton-Radek, K. (2004). *Sleep quality in young adults.* New York: Mellon Press.

WEB SITES

National Sleep Foundation. http://www.sleepfoundation.org. Best-known nonprofit foundation for sleep.

Restless Legs Foundation. http://www.rls.org

Sleepnet.com. http://www.sleepnet.com. General practical information about sleep. This site includes information for the public as well as sleep clinician links.

Simplified Classification of Sleep Disorders

Sleep disorder	Summary description of disorder
Insomnia	Difficulty in initiating and / or maintaining sleep occurring 3 or more nights per week and persisting for at least 6 months. Possible daytime mood and performance effects.
Normal aging	Developmentally normal changes in sleep and wakefulness.
Sleep-Related Breathing Disorder (SBD)	Cessation of breathing (apnea), loud snoring, choking / fighting for breath during sleep. Morning headache, dry mouth, obesity, excessive daytime sleepiness / involuntary naps may present.
Periodic Limb Movements in Sleep (PLMS) and Restless Legs Syndrome (RLS)	Motor restlessness during sleep and relaxation, involuntary limb movements. Associated with insomnia and/or excessive daytime sleepiness.
Circadian Rhythm Sleep Disorders	Chronobiological disorders involving misalignment between sleep pattern and local time. Delayed or advanced sleep phases produce complaints of insomnia and / or excessive sleepiness.
Narcolepsy	Irresistible sleep attacks at inappropriate times. Sometimes with cataplexy (loss of muscle tone triggered by emotion), hypnagogic hallucinations, sleep paralysis, and disturbed nighttime sleep.
Parasomnias	Abnormal behaviors in NREM sleep (e.g., sleepwalking, sleep bruxism) and REM sleep (e.g., nightmares) and in transition between wakefulness and sleep (e.g., sleep talking).
Sleep Disorders Associated with Medical / Psychiatric Disorders	A wide range of disorders involves sleep symptomatology. Neurologic disorders (e.g., dementia, Parkinson's disease), other medical disorders (e.g., cardiac ischemia, pulmonary disease, gastrointestinal problems), and mental disorders (e.g., affective disorders, alcoholism).
Extrinsic Sleep Disorders	A wide range of exogenous causes. Includes hypnotic-, alcohol-, and stimulant-dependency sleep disorder.

Source: Based on the revised International Classification of Sleep Disorders, American Sleep Disorders Association, 2004.

ACCREDITED SLEEP CENTERS

To find a sleep center in your area, go to the American Academy of Sleep Medicine Web site at http://www.aasmnet.org

RELAXATION SCRIPTS

EXAMPLE 1

Before you retire to bed, make sure that your bedroom is free of tension and worry. You will prepare yourself for relaxation and slumber by quietly freeing yourself from television or newspapers as you focus your attention and strength on winding down from your day. Intuitively, you will begin to turn off lights and quiet your mind. As you get into bed, you will automatically begin to relax. Your breathing will become deeply and profoundly relaxed and methodical. You will notice how you intuitively begin to fall asleep. You can rest assured that your body knows how to fall asleep and stay asleep and rest. You will be surprised at how well you are able to fall deeply asleep. You will be able to sleep through the night and awake refreshed and rested for the day. Your body will welcome the rest, as it is able to benefit from deep sleep. You will notice how easily you adapt to good, restful sleep. You have confidence in knowing that as you sleep, your body is building strength and building its immune system. You will be able to know how profoundly your body is able to benefit from deep, deep sleep.

EXAMPLE 2

Imagine walking toward your bedroom, and as you are walking you are giving yourself permission to leave all worries, concerns, or anything that is troubling you outside of your bedroom. When you awaken in the morning, you can retrieve these worries, concerns, or troubles when you walk out of your bedroom. There is no need to bring these with you because your bedroom is a safe haven. It is your personal safety zone. It is here that you can experience comfort, safety, and peace.

You notice the bedroom door is getting closer and closer, and you are feeling more and more relaxed and peaceful. There is nothing of concern to you as approach your bedroom, and this feeling of relaxation becomes deeper and deeper, especially as you walk into your bedroom. You notice that you are feeling calmer, more secure, and more peaceful as you approach your bed. Your limbs are growing heavier and heavier as you pull back the covers of your bed. As you get into bed, you notice how comfortable you feel lying in your bed. Your mind is quiet, and you feel calm and relaxed. Your eyelids are beginning to get heavier and heavier, and you welcome this feeling.

When you are ready, your eyelids close. You are lying in comfort and notice that you are free of any emotional or physical discomfort. You do not have any concerns because your mind is very quiet and calm. You are feeling sleepier and sleepier. There is no need to check the clock because your body knows how to fall asleep, how to stay asleep, and how to wake up when it is ready to wake up. The clock is unimportant, and you will not feel a need to look at it because you are working with your body, nature's original sleep-wake clock. It is important to remember that when your body is ready to sleep, it will sleep. This experience of sleep will be a deep and profound sleep. If you awaken during the night, you will easily return to sleep, even if you have gotten up to use the bathroom, because your body knows how to sleep. You feel peaceful and safe and are very, very sleepy. You know that your body knows how to sleep because you have done it since you were a child. And much like a child, you welcome sleep, and your body will wake when it has had enough sleep. It is important to sleep just long enough and to keep the same bedtimes and wake times, even during weekends. Rest assured, you will sleep well. You have the ability to master deep restorative sleep, just as you have the ability to manage the day-to-day activities of your life right now. When you wake to your alarm in the morning, you will feel refreshed and energetic and ready to start your day.

Index

About the Authors

KATHY SEXTON-RADEK, PhD, CBSM, is professor of psychology at Elmhurst College and Director of Psychological Services, Suburban Pulmonary and Sleep Associates in Illinois. She is the author of numerous peer-reviewed articles, book chapters, and books in the areas of sleep medicine, pain management, behavioral medicine, and health psychology. She serves on the Public Relations Committee of the Behavioral Section of the American Association of Sleep Medicine. She is also a member of the American Psychological Association, the Illinois Counseling Association, the Association for Behavioral and Cognitive Therapy, and the Sleep Research Society.

GINA GRACI, PhD, CBSM, is a licensed clinical psychologist and sleep specialist. She received her PhD from the University of North Texas and is a certified behavioral sleep medicine specialist with the American Academy of Sleep Medicine. She has a clinical practice in Chicago and is a research investigator at the Chicago Research Center. Dr. Graci has conducted clinical trials concerning sleep and oncology with funding from both the private and public sectors. She has also presented and published widely in leading medical journals and has been frequently interviewed for stories in national and local print and broadcast media.

PHYLLIS C. ZEE, MD, PhD, is an associate professor of neurology and neurobiology and the director of the Sleep Disorders Center at Northwestern Memorial Hospital and the associate director of the Center for Circadian Biology and Medicine at Northwestern University.